Co

F
burning
Diet

This book has been compiled with the assistance of
hundreds of brand-name manufacturers. Other sources are listed on
pages 64-5.

HarperCollins Publishers
Westerhill Road, Bishopbriggs, Glasgow G64 2QT

www.collins.co.uk

First published 2007

Reprint 10 9 8 7 6 5 4 3 2 1 0

© HarperCollins Publishers 2007

ISBN 10 0-00-723235-7
ISBN 13 978-0-00-723235-2

All rights reserved. Collins Gem® is a registered
trademark of HarperCollinsPublishers Limited

Editorial by Grapevine Publishing Services, London
Text by Kate Santon
Design by Judith Ash

Printed in Italy by Amadeus S.r.l.

CONTENTS

INTRODUCTION

People have always looked for the dieting equivalent of the Holy Grail; a diet that works, is easy to follow and one that makes it possible to keep the weight off afterwards. Fad diets come and go but for the most part making no difference. Calorie counting is the old standby but can get boring, leave you hungry and not help keep your weight down in the long-term. It's all too easy to put weight back on when you stop weighing and measuring. Eating particular foods becomes antisocial and tedious, whether you're consuming lots of fibre or lots of cabbage soup, and meal-replacement plans bore. There have been many kinds of temporary, short-term diet plans but they aren't, usually, long-term solutions because they don't go any further. However, some diets have lasted rather longer and have been modified and adapted as the understanding of the way the body works has changed and developed.

The first high-protein diet to attract attention was Dr Robert Atkins 'Atkins

Diet', publicised in his book *Diet Revolution* in 1972. It turned all received wisdom upside-down, suggesting that you eliminate carbohydrates – bread, sugar, rice, pasta, fruit, potatoes and most vegetables – completely. Atkins dieters concentrated on protein, and high-fat protein at that. They could eat all the meat, eggs, cream, fat and butter they wanted. For many people this sounded too good to be true, and the medical establishment was horrified, worrying that such an extreme diet, heavy in saturated fats, might cause strokes, heart disease, kidney disorders, osteoporosis, even malnutrition. Some dieters did suffer, usually from bad breath and constipation, but there were also a few suggestions of longer-term problems. However, many people also lost weight.

In the meantime, medical research was inviting more and more emphasis to be placed on the need for foodstuffs to be low in fat. Low-fat products were developed, low-fat diets were commonplace but people didn't get any thinner. In fact, overall obesity levels rose to such an extent that governments began to worry about the consequences.

The Atkins Diet began a new surge in popularity at the end of the 1990s, in a modified form. It still concentrated on proteins but allowed some non-starchy carbs, though the introductory phase cut most of them out. The aim was to get the body to burn fat for the fuel it needed, entering a state known as ketosis. Again dieters tended to have bad breath from the ketosis, constipation and a general feeling of ill health; some reported headaches, confusion and dizziness, though many of these effects were attributed to people either remaining on the introductory phase for too long or not drinking enough water. A few deaths were even alleged to have been caused by the diet. It began to fall out of popularity and there was a lot of negative publicity. However, many Atkins dieters were also losing weight, often very quickly and dramatically. Something interesting did seem to be happening, despite the problems.

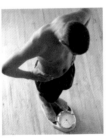

Gradually more moderate diets began to appear, 'higher in protein' rather than 'high protein', 'low-carb' rather than 'no carb'. They don't insist on enormous quantities of protein at the expense of everything else and they are – by and large – discriminating about the type of protein. The emphasis is now on proteins that are lower in saturated fats, like skinless chicken, meat which is not only trimmed of visible fat but is leaner as well, and fish, particularly the oily fish which are high in Omega-3 fatty acids. In most of the new diets, and in all of them once out of any demanding introductory phases, proteins are combined with carbs. They concentrate on the 'right' carbs and often use the glycaemic index of carbs (or net carbs, in the case of Atkins) – a measure of how quickly they are digested – to determine which are the ones to choose. Regulating blood-sugar levels is seen to be critical, something which these diets have in common with the other major diet trend at the beginning of the 21st century, the GI diets.

Blood sugar and insulin

Carbohydrates have a direct and marked effect on blood sugar. When you eat a slice of bread, your body uses the digestible carbs it contains to form glucose, a simple sugar. This is very rapidly absorbed into the bloodstream and provides the body with energy. Glucose is the major fuel for most of the tissues in the body and so is regulated by complex mechanisms that ensure it doesn't plummet too low or soar too high. Increased glucose levels stimulate the production of insulin in the pancreas as insulin enables glucose to enter the cells of the body, making it possible for them to use it for energy. As the level of insulin rises, glucose is removed from the blood into the cells. As the cells absorb glucose, blood-sugar levels fall away, and then so do insulin levels. Excess glucose is stored as glycogen in the muscles or liver, or converted to fat.

If you eat something containing quickly digested carbs, such as a chocolate bar that is high in sugar, insulin floods your body in response, which ultimately pushes glucose levels too low. Your body now needs more glucose and sends out signals – hunger, mainly – to tell you so and prompt you to provide it, maybe in the form of another bar of chocolate. It's a roller-coaster with highs and lows but it can be turned into a more stable process which is much better for your health – and for your weight loss. The problem lies in the high level of refined, easily digested carbs which is a normal feature of the modern Western diet, so reducing those – or cutting them out as close to completely as possible – is vital.

Slowly digested carbs, such as those in whole grains and pulses, smooth out the ups and downs. Blood-sugar levels, and therefore insulin levels, rise and fall much more gradually; the peaks and troughs are less

The Glucose Process

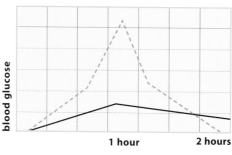

blood glucose

1 hour   2 hours

- - - - Easily digested carbs
———— Slowly digested carbs

extreme. Not only are you putting much less stress on your body, but it may also take much longer for you to become hungry again. Protein, together with fat, has a vital role to play in normalising insulin levels by slowing down the rate at which carbs are absorbed. Replacing the refined carbs with healthier ones and extra, healthier protein is good for your health and for losing weight.

Another advantage of eating more protein is that it helps to control hunger pangs. Foods high in protein

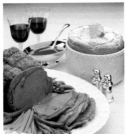

have a high 'satiety value': they keep you feeling satisfied for longer. Not only is this useful immediately, reducing the need for snacking (which would elevate both blood-sugar levels and calorie intake) but it also makes sticking to a diet easier and can turn it into a way of life, rather than a temporary solution.

In addition, there is some evidence that cutting back on refined carbs and replacing them with protein boosts the levels of HDL, the good type of blood cholesterol. It also seems to lower the level of blood triglycerides – and high levels are associated with an increased risk of heart disease.

Ketosis
Some high-protein diets stress yet another possible advantage of smoothing out the blood-sugar roller-coaster. High levels of insulin encourage the body to store excess glucose as fat. Low insulin levels encourage the body to release that, making it

available as a source of energy, sometimes described as your body 'burning fat'. Ketones are released when this is happening and can be detected on the breath – hence the halitosis that some dieters have reported – and in the urine. The Atkins Diet suggests that you test your urine, although the testing sticks only register the presence of one type of ketone.

It should be noted that some specialists have reservations about whether inducing the state of ketosis is actually desirable or necessary for weight loss. Not all of the new high-protein diets see it as essential; in fact, some regard it as a sign that you've gone too far.

If you are overweight but healthy, ketosis shouldn't generally be problematic but it can be for people with kidney problems or those who are on anti-hypertension medication because it is associated with some dehydration and a general decrease in fluid volume in the body. All high-protein diets, old and new, stress the importance of drinking enough water. You should always check with your doctor before embarking on a serious weight-loss programme; this is vital if you have any kind of chronic illness. Strict high-protein diets are definitely unsuitable for people with kidney problems.

WHAT SHOULD YOU BE EATING?

Fad diets, diets that exclude some types of food or that require dieters to concentrate on a specific food like grapefruit, never address the basic problem: the way of eating that led to weight gain in the first place. What is needed is a diet that provides realistic, long-term change, and does so relatively painlessly and in a healthy way. The new high-protein diets are less limiting than earlier versions, they burn fat efficiently so helping your weight-loss efforts, and they provide a way of eating that can become a way of life. The best of them recognise that the body needs fats, carbs, vitamins and minerals as well as protein.

Protein

Proteins are vital for building, growing and developing every part of your body. Muscles and vital organs are made up of protein; bones are made of it; every single process in your body requires it. Proteins have two main functions. They promote growth and form the framework of the body's main structures like skin, hair and nails – a constant supply is needed for running repairs – and they maintain the supplies of hormones, enzymes and antibodies which regulate many of the body's most important functions, like the ability to digest food.

Strangely, protein has been studied much less than fats or carbs but this is beginning to change; one recent consequence is that the importance of soya protein has been recognised.

Amino acids are protein's building blocks. The body can make some of them but others, called 'essential' amino acids, have to come from food. Proteins are divided into 'complete' and 'incomplete' proteins according to whether they supply all the essential amino acids. Those from animal sources – fish, meat, eggs, dairy – are complete proteins, as is soya.

Eggs fell out of favour and it was common for diets to recommend cutting egg consumption because of the cholesterol they contain. Some writers still suggest using only the whites. Eggs are, however, a valuable source of many nutrients, and there has never been any research clearly demonstrating that people who eat a lot of eggs are more prone to heart attacks than those who only eat a few. There is general agreement among dietitians and scientists that eating an egg a day is not harmful for most people, and many of the new high-protein diets include eggs.

Soya is being recommended more and more, as the evidence of the benefits it provides increases, with many of the new diets suggesting tofu – made from soya – as one of your regular sources of protein. There are various kinds available, and a good selection can often be found in supermarkets and health-food shops as well as oriental stores (where it may be called bean curd). It might be worth considering organic tofu, however, as soya is one of the most common crops to be genetically modified.

Plant proteins are incomplete but, providing you eat a good variety of nuts and seeds, and wholegrains and legumes (beans, chickpeas, split peas and lentils), they can supply the amino acids you need. These are, however, frequently high in carbs and/or calories and eating too many of them can blow your diet. Most of the new high-protein diets require you to monitor your carb levels, so if you are vegetarian you may need to look at other sources of protein – check out Rose Elliot's *Vegetarian Low-Carb Diet* or Barry Sears' *The Soy Zone* for suggestions. All protein has a steady, gentle effect on blood sugar, avoiding the steep rises and falls.

Fats

When high-protein diets first became popular, one of the main reasons why medics were concerned was the inclusion of substantial amounts of all types of fat. The new high-protein diets are much lower in the saturated fats that gave rise to such concern. All fats are not alike, so it is important to choose those that are best for you.

Fat is actually necessary. The body uses it for many processes, from manufacturing hormones to enabling the absorption of fat-soluble vitamins. Like protein, fats in the diet slow down the rate at which food is absorbed, helping to moderate the highs and lows in blood-sugar levels. They also give food a lot of its taste, which is one of the factors that makes you feel satisfied after a meal, so choosing the right ones is critical.

Dietary fat is divided into two main categories – saturated and unsaturated. Saturated fat is generally solid at

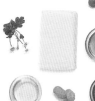

room temperature and often comes from animal sources – butter, lard, the white fat on meat, cream, cheese – though coconut and palm oils are also high in saturates. They're often used in processed food like biscuits, pies and crisps; deep-fried food is often cooked in saturated fat. These fats have been associated with higher rates of blocked arteries, leading to strokes and heart attacks, and most of the newer diets suggest they should be eaten in moderation.

Trans fats, sometimes called hydrogenated fats, should be avoided completely if possible. These lurk in biscuits, cakes, some spreads and margarines, some breads and fast foods. They are linked to high cholesterol levels and increased rates of heart disease so check labels. Most manufacturers are trying to cut trans fats from their products.

Unsaturated fats are the ones to go for. These are liquid at room temperature and can be divided into three types:
• Monounsaturated fats – found in olive, groundnut and rapeseed oils and spreads, walnuts and avocados. They have a beneficial effect on the heart.
• Omega-3 polyunsaturated fats – found in oily fish like salmon, mackerel, herring, tuna and sardines; in

linseed, wheatgerm, sesame seed, soya beans, grain-fed chickens' eggs, evening primrose oil, olive and rapeseed oils. They help to thin the blood and are necessary for brain function.

• Omega-6 polyunsaturated fats – found in vegetable, sunflower and corn oils, soya margarines and sun-flower spreads. They don't have the health benefits of the Omega-3 fats but are better than saturated fats and trans fats.

The newer high-protein diets vary in their advice about whether dieters should monitor their levels of fat intake closely or not. However, they are united in stressing the importance of using predominantly unsaturated fats.

Carbohydrates

Carbs are found mostly in plant foods, like fruit and vegetables, beans, grains, lentils, and in products derived from them, like breakfast cereals, bread or pasta. Cutting them out completely could lead to health problems, a fact recognised by the new high-protein diets. There are some carbs which should be eliminated as much as possible – refined, easily digested carbs. Refined carbs will make your blood sugar shoot up and give you few benefits in exchange. Less-refined carbs are high in fibre,

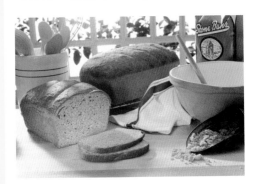

necessary for the digestion, and also contain important micronutrients, like the B vitamins. Some of the new high-protein diets reduce carbs drastically during an introductory phase. Others do not but most require you to monitor the quantity you eat. As a broad guideline, and bearing in mind the diet you choose to follow, you should go for:

- wholegrain breads, high-fibre cereals, wholemeal pasta and brown rice
- pulses – beans, lentils, chickpeas, etc.
- vegetables – except starchy ones like potatoes, beets and parsnips
- whole fresh fruit – except bananas, which are high in carbs and should be eaten in moderation.

You should avoid processed and refined carbs:
- white flour and anything made from it, including bread, cakes and non-wholemeal pasta
- sugar and foods with a high sugar content, such as fizzy drinks, sweets and many ready meals
- rice, especially easy-cook varieties
- refined cereals (non-wholegrain)
- potatoes, beets and starchy vegetables
- fruit juices.

All these will cause blood-sugar spikes. The more 'whole' something is, the more gently it will affect your blood sugar. Sweetness is a useful guide too – foods which are immediately sweet to the taste are likely to be no-nos.

The fibre in carbs is important. It keeps your digestive system working properly, relieving constipation. It protects against diverticulitis and colon cancer, and there is some evidence that it reduces the risk of bowel cancer. Some diets recommend using psyllium (available in health-food shops) to maintain adequate fibre levels, but including enough vegetables and unrefined carbs in your diet should also do the trick and bring additional benefits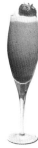

from the vitamins and minerals they include. The lack of dietary fibre and lowered levels of some B vitamins were two of the worries the health profession had about early high-protein diets.

Vitamins and Minerals

Proteins, fats and carbs are the big three nutrients but there are many other 'micronutrients' which are just as essential. A good, well-balanced diet should ensure that you get everything you need but adding a multivitamin and mineral supplement is recommended in the introductory phases of some diets. Concerns have been expressed in the past about high-protein diets not providing enough of some of the B vitamins, especially vitamin B1, and folic acid but this should not be so much of a problem on the newer ones.

Check that you regularly eat foods containing all of the vitamins and minerals listed on pages 25 to 27. If you decide to take a supplement, then don't exceed the RDA (recommended daily allowance) given on the packaging as some can be dangerous in high doses. Avoid any supplements that are close to their sell-by date as they will be less potent. Vegetarians may need to supplement their diets with vitamin B12, which cannot be obtained from non-animal foods.

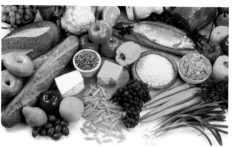

Vitamin A: Eggs, butter, fish oils, dark green and yellow fruits and vegetables, liver. *Essential for:* strong bones, good eyesight, healthy skin, healing.

Vitamin B1 (*Thiamine*): Plant and animal foods, especially wholegrain products, brown rice, seafood and beans. *Essential for:* growth, nerve function, conversion of blood sugar into energy.

Vitamin B2 (*Riboflavin*): Milk and dairy produce, green leafy vegetables, liver, kidneys, yeast. *Essential for:* cell growth and reproduction, energy production.

Vitamin B3 (*Niacin*): Meats, fish and poultry, wholegrains, peanuts and avocados. *Essential for:* digestion, energy, the nervous system.

Vitamin B5 (*Pantothenic acid*): Organ meats, fish, eggs, chicken, nuts and wholegrain cereals. *Essential for:* strengthening immunity and fighting infections, healing wounds.

Vitamin B6 (*Pyridoxine*): Meat, eggs, wholegrains, yeast, cabbage, melon, molasses. *Essential for:* the production of new cells, a healthy immune system, production of antibodies and white blood cells.

Vitamin B12 (*Cyanocobalamin*): Fish, dairy produce, beef, pork, lamb, organ meats, eggs and milk.

Essential for: energy and concentration, production of red blood cells, growth in children.

Vitamin C: Fresh fruit and vegetables, potatoes, leafy herbs and berries.

Essential for: healthy skin, bones, muscles, healing, eyesight and protection from viruses.

Vitamin D: Milk and dairy produce, eggs, fatty fish.

Essential for: healthy teeth and bones, vital for growth.

Vitamin E: Nuts, seeds, eggs, milk, wholegrains, leafy green vegetables, avocados and soya.

Essential for: absorption of iron and essential fatty acids, slowing the ageing process, increasing fertility.

Vitamin K: Green vegetables, milk products, apricots, wholegrains, cod liver oil.

Essential for: blood clotting.

Calcium: Dairy produce, leafy green vegetables, salmon, nuts, root vegetables, tofu.

Essential for: strong bones and teeth, hormones and muscles, blood clotting and the regulation of blood pressure.

Iron: Liver, kidney, cocoa powder, dark chocolate, shellfish, pulses, dark green vegetables, egg yolks, red meat, beans, molasses.

Essential for: supply of oxygen to the cells and healthy immune system.

Magnesium: Brown rice, soya beans, nuts, wholegrains, bitter chocolate, legumes.

Essential for: transmission of

nerve impulses, development of bones, growth and repair of cells.

Potassium: Avocados, leafy green vegetables, bananas, fruit and vegetable juices, potatoes and nuts.

Essential for: maintaining water balance, nerve and muscle function.

Chromium: Liver, whole grains, meat and cheese, brewer's yeast, mushrooms, egg yolk.

Essential for: stimulating insulin. Chromium also governs the 'glucose tolerance factor' which is often not working properly in failed dieters.

Iodine: Fish and seafood,

pineapple, dairy produce, raisins.

Essential for: keeping hair, skin, nails and teeth healthy.

Folic acid: Fruit, green leafy vegetables, nuts, pulses, yeast extracts.

Essential for: production of new cells (working with vitamin B12) and is especially important during pregnancy to prevent birth defects.

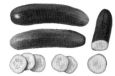

Calcium

Calcium isn't just the main mineral component of bones, nails and teeth; it has many other important functions including aiding the digestion of food. There's a potential problem with high-protein diets because the more protein you eat, the more calcium your body needs to digest it. If it doesn't have enough, it will draw calcium from its reserve – the skeleton. If you eat high levels of protein for a short period of time – for example, during the introductory phase of a classic high-protein diet – then you probably won't do any long-term damage but research is continuing. This is another reason why you should not stay too long on the introductory phase of any high-protein diet, particularly the more restrictive ones.

Try to ensure that your calcium intake is adequate – check the sources on page 26 – and consider whether you need to supplement it. One thing to note is that not all the calcium in food is digested, and dairy products in particular contain components which aid

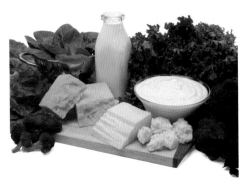

absorption. If you are lactose-intolerant you may still be able to eat yoghurt and cheese; if you use soya milk, be sure to buy a brand fortified with calcium. Vegetarians seem to absorb and retain more calcium than meat-eaters, so calcium deficiency shouldn't be too much of a problem if you don't eat meat.

READING LABELS

It is impossible to avoid all packaged foods, no matter how strenuously some diets may recommend that you should. Some products can be ruled out fairly painlessly and you can help yourself by being aware of what you are buying by using the ingredient lists and nutritional information on the packaging.

Ingredients are listed in descending order, so if sugar is listed first, then there is more sugar in the product than anything else. Sugar can go under many names, so look out for corn syrup, fructose, lactose, glucose, sucrose, maltose, dextrose, galactose, malto-dextrin, levulose – and don't forget honey. Watch the fats: trans fats, which you should avoid, may be called hydrogenated or partially hydrogenated fats. Lots of things you don't recognise – E numbers, preservatives, artificial colours and flavourings – are a sign of a heavily processed food which is probably best left on the supermarket shelf.

The nutritional information isn't always clear but can provide good guidelines. Go for foods with the highest fibre count when comparing products. Always check the 'per 100g' figures; portion sizes can vary enormously, may be unrealistically small and they don't provide a valid comparison between one product with another. For your overall health, you should also think about salt when reading labels. It is usually listed as sodium and you have to multiply it by 2.5 to get the quantity of salt. As a quick guide, 0.5g of sodium per 100g is too much.

Finally, beware of nutrition flashes like 'low fat' or 'low sugar' as they can be misleading:

- 'Fat free' means a food that contains less than 0.15g fat per 100g but '90% fat free' means it has 10% fat. 'Virtually fat free' means it has less than 0.3g of fat per 100g; 'low fat' means it must have 3g or less per 100g. 'Reduced fat' means there's 25% less fat than in the standard equivalent.
- 'No added sugar' means sugar hasn't been added during manufacture, not that the product has no sugar in it at all. 'Unsweetened' means that no sugar or sweetener has been added.
- 'Reduced salt' has no legal definition. The Food Standards Agency say that foods labelled 'reduced salt' should have 25% less salt than a normal equivalent.

Finally, try to consider the whole picture: low-fat products may be high in sugars, for example, and a vitamin-enriched product might contain E numbers.

HOW MUCH DO YOU NEED TO LOSE?

Everyone is different, so there are no hard and fast rules about how much you should weigh. Consider your overall build; if you have a naturally large frame, you'll never turn yourself into a tiny person. Everyone has a genetic predisposition for a particular weight range. The most traditional way of seeing how much weight you need to lose is to use a height and weight chart, like the one on pages 32-3.

Nowadays the body mass index (BMI) is frequently used. This is a way of assessing how much fat you're carrying. If you are very muscular (muscles weigh more than fat), or pregnant, then this wouldn't apply, but neither would the height and weight charts. To find out your BMI, divide your weight in kilograms by the square of your height in metres (it's easier than it sounds): weight ÷ (height x height) = BMI. For example, if you are 1.65m tall (5ft 5in) and weigh 76kg (12st), it would work out like this:

1.65 x 1.65 = 2.72
76 ÷ 2.72 = 27.94

Tables for Standard Body Weight

Men

Height m (ft)	Small Frame kg (lbs)	Medium Frame kg (lbs)	Large Frame kg (lbs)
1.55 (5'1")	49–59 (107–130)	51–61 (113–134)	55–64 (121–140)
1.57 (5'2")	50–60 (110–132)	53–63 (116–138)	56–65 (124–144)
1.60 (5'3")	51–61 (113–134)	54–64 (119–140)	58–68 (127–150)
1.63 (5'4")	53–61 (116–135)	55–65 (122–142)	59–70 (131–154)
1.65 (5'5")	54–62 (119–137)	57–66 (125–146)	60–72 (133–159)
1.68 (5'6")	56–64 (123–140)	59–68 (129–149)	62–74 (137–163)
1.70 (5'7")	58–65 (127–143)	60–69 (133–152)	64–76 (142–167)
1.73 (5'8")	60–66 (131–145)	62–71 (137–155)	66–78 (146–171)
1.75 (5'9")	61–68 (135–149)	64–72 (141–158)	68–80 (150–175)
1.78 (5'10")	63–69 (139–152)	66–73 (145–161)	70–81 (154–179)
1.80 (5'11")	65–70 (143–155)	68–75 (149–165)	72–83 (159–183)
1.83 (6')	67–72 (147–159)	70–77 (153–169)	74–85 (163–187)
1.85 (6'1")	69–75 (151–165)	71–80 (157–175)	76–86 (167–189)
1.88 (6'2")	70–76 (155–168)	73–81 (161–179)	78–89 (171–197)
1.90 (6'3")	72–79 (157–173)	75–84 (166–185)	80–92 (176–202)

Women

Height m (ft)	Small Frame kg (lbs)	Medium Frame kg (lbs)	Large Frame kg (lbs)
1.47 (4'10")	41–49 (91–108)	43–52 (95–115)	47–54 (103–119)
1.50 (4'11")	42–51 (93–112)	44–55 (98–121)	48–57 (106–125)
1.52 (5')	44–52 (96–115)	46–57 (101–124)	49–58 (109–128)
1.55 (5'1")	45–54 (99–118)	47–58 (104–127)	51–59 (112–131)
1.57 (5'2")	46–55 (102–121)	49–60 (107–132)	52–61 (115–135)
1.60 (5'3")	48–56 (105–124)	50–62 (110–135)	54–63 (118–138)
1.63 (5'4")	49–58 (108–127)	51–63 (113–138)	55–65 (122–142)
1.65 (5'5")	50–59 (111–130)	53–64 (117–141)	57–66 (126–145)
1.68 (5'6")	52–60 (115–133)	55–66 (121–144)	59–67 (130–148)
1.70 (5'7")	54–62 (119–136)	57–67 (125–147)	61–69 (134–151)
1.73 (5'8")	56–63 (123–139)	58–68 (128–150)	62–71 (137–155)
1.75 (5'9")	58–64 (127–142)	60–69 (133–153)	64–73 (141–159)
1.78 (5'10")	59–66 (131–145)	62–71 (137–156)	66–75 (146–165)
1.80 (5'11")	61–68 (135–148)	64–72 (141–159)	68–77 (150–170)
1.83 (6')	63–69 (138–151)	65–74 (143–163)	69–79 (153–173)

BMI figures are grouped into categories, so check to see where your score fits on the scale:

- less than 15   emaciated
- 15–19   underweight
- 19–25   average
- 25–30   overweight
- 30–40   obese
- over 40   severely obese

These BMI 'cut-offs' apply to healthy adults, but not to people with some specific medical conditions, anyone pregnant or elderly, or anyone under 18. The BMI's broad general guidelines are useful and you should certainly see your doctor if your BMI falls into the emaciated or obese range as you could be damaging your health.

The right weight for you is one at which you feel comfortable, energetic and, above all else, healthy. Once you've got a BMI of between 19 and 25, you're at a healthy weight, so use the BMI to give yourself a rough target. Multiply your height in metres squared times the BMI you want to achieve (say, 25) to find your ideal weight: (height x height) x 25 = ideal weight in kg. How much do you need to lose? Setting a realistic and achievable target is essential.

You should always consult your doctor before
starting to diet if:

- you have had a stroke or have a chronic condition
  like heart disease
- you take any regular medication
- you're pregnant
- you are over 40 and have more than 5kg to lose
- you're planning to start exercising too, but haven't
  done so for ages.

Exercise

If you take in more calories in the form of food than
you use in the form of energy, you put weight on.
Raising your metabolic rate will help you use more

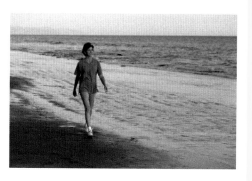

calories, and exercise is a vital part of successful weight-loss plans, high-protein or not. All the new high-protein diets stress the importance of exercise and some give instructions for easy exercises. Think about increasing the amount of exercise you take every day – get off the bus a stop early and walk, park far away from the supermarket entrance – as well as adding a specific activity to your routine. Exercise doesn't have to mean a gym workout or traditional sport; a salsa or line-dancing class provides a good alternative, for example.

WHY CHOOSE ONE OF THE NEW HIGH-PROTEIN DIETS?

Earlier versions of the high-protein diet were extreme and quite possibly unhealthy but did produce some interesting results, helping dieters to lose weight relatively easily. The new ones are much more balanced and – providing you're basically healthy, don't spend too long in the introductory phase and drink enough water – they should do you no harm.

Hunger shouldn't be a problem, and these diets shouldn't be boring, either. They are, by and large, flexible enough to integrate into daily life – you can even incorporate eating out with some care (see pages 219–34). While it is important to lose weight slowly and steadily in order to keep it off, many people need the encouragement of early weight loss, and that should be possible on most of the new high-protein diets. Any initial quick weight loss should settle down to a much steadier rate.

It is important to make sure the diet you choose suits your lifestyle, as well as being safe. Think about questions like:

· Will it fit into your daily routines?
· Do you want to be flexible or are you happy to rely on meal plans?

Then consider:

· Does the diet provide a balanced selection of food?
· Are any healthy foods – fruit, for instance – permanently excluded?
· What is forbidden in the introductory phase and how long does it last?
· Is everything explained fully?
· Does it seem to be advocating anything 'cranky'? If it relies on a lot of supplements, for example, it might be deficient in nutrients.
· Does it promise rapid weight loss? This may not be a good sign – to have any chance of

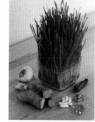

maintaining your new weight, you need to lose most of your excess gradually.

- Does the diet discuss and address potential problems?
- Finally, your diet needs to become a way of life, so check that there's enough information on how to keep your new figure once you've achieved it.

Don't try and make up your own high-protein diet from scratch. You are retraining your body and need to get it right; you can improvise later once you understand the principles through seeing them work. Check out some of the following high-protein diets and find one that suits you instead. Once again, though, if you have a problem with your kidneys, you should not really be following a high-protein diet – talk to your doctor.

CSIRO TOTAL WELLBEING DIET: DR MANNY NOAKES WITH DR PETER CLIFTON

The Commonwealth Scientific and Research Organisation is Australia's national science agency and both authors work for CSIRO Health Sciences and Nutrition. The diet is based on controlled scientific trials, which led to the development of a 'protein-plus eating plan'. This was partly funded by Dairy Australia and Meat & Livestock Australia, has been thoroughly tested on volunteers and on members of the public through *Australian Women's Weekly*.

There is no separate introductory phase but it isn't a one-diet-fits-all scheme. You choose a level to match your gender and how active you are (you are shown how to calculate your energy requirements), so if you are a very active man you may eat more than an inactive woman would. If you are losing weight too rapidly, and feeling hungry, you move up a level. Most women will probably start on level 1, men on level 3. There is a maintenance plan to follow once you've reached your target, and plenty of information on exercise.

Foods are divided into units, and eating the recommended units gives you a balanced diet. The stress is on lean protein, 'good' carbs and low-fat dairy products, and the authors recommend sticking to the day-by-day menu plans – enough are provided for 12 weeks – for the first few weeks at least, while you get used to the diet. These plans are based on level 1 and – within guidelines – there can be substitutions but you must eat the protein allowance as foods rich in protein provide many important nutrients, help you to feel satisfied for longer and control blood fats. Checklists and shopping lists are provided to keep you on track, and there is nutritional information so you understand why you are being asked to make certain choices.

YOUR DAILY ALLOWANCE, AT LEVEL 1:
Lean protein: 2 units for dinner, 1 for lunch.
1 unit = 100g raw weight of protein food. For dinner, chicken is recommended for one night a week, fish for two and red meat (beef, lamb or veal) for four nights. The lunch unit can be any protein, or two eggs or an extra dairy unit.   You must eat the protein foods each day.
Wholegrain bread: 2 units a day
1 unit = a 35g slice. If you like, one of these units can be substituted with: 2 crispbreads; a medium potato; a third of a cup of cooked rice, noodles, beans or lentils; or half a cup of cooked pasta (Australian 'cups' are 250ml, bigger than an American cup measure).
High-fibre cereal: 1 unit a day
40g of any high-fibre cereal, like All-Bran, or a slice of wholegrain toast instead

Dairy: 2 units a day
1 unit is either 250ml low-fat milk, 200g low-fat yoghurt, 200g low-fat custard or dairy dessert, 25g cheddar or full-fat cheese, 50g reduced-fat cheese
Fruit: 2 units a day
1 unit = 150g fresh fruit or unsweetened tinned fruit
Vegetables: 2.5 units a day
1 unit = 1 cup cooked veg, chosen from an extensive list. The authors recommend that the half unit should be salad.
Fats and oils: 3 units a day
1 unit = 1 tsp liquid oil, 3 tsp soft margarine, 60g avocado, or 20g nuts and seeds.
Optional
250ml of low-calorie soup per day, and two 150ml glasses of wine each week (or any snack food with the same calorie value as the wine, but only once a week).

Once you reach your target you begin to add more food, while still following the guidelines: lean or low-fat protein at each meal, wholegrain breads and cereals, eating regular meals, always having breakfast and planning your snacks (these are only regularly included at maintenance level).

Sample menus

Breakfast

2 slices of wholegrain toast with light margarine, plus
200g yoghurt; one poached, boiled or scrambled egg
with half a tomato and mushrooms; or high-fibre
breakfast cereal with low-fat milk and a sliced banana.

Lunch

Tuna with cannellini bean and basil salad; beef and
vegetable soup with a slice of wholegrain bread and
50g low-fat cheese; or salmon salad with tarragon
and caper dressing.

Dinner

Spiced lamb chops with ratatouille followed by a
low-fat dairy dessert; swordfish steaks with warm
zucchini and olive salad followed by stewed rhubarb;
or char-grilled beef fillet with mushrooms and
caramelised onion, followed by fresh fruit.

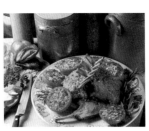

Effectiveness

As long as you can
stick to the diet
and are willing to
do so completely,
there is no reason
why you should
not lose weight on
it. If you are in a

position to plan your meals well in advance, the structure of the CSIRO diet is ideal; if you are more independent you might find it difficult to follow successfully. There are many recipes, and though some measurements are Australian, they are easily adapted. You may also need to make substitutions because some ingredients may be unfamiliar or unavailable in the UK. Kilojoules are used rather than the calories more familiar to UK dieters (there are 4.18 calories to the kilojoule) but so long as you don't try and convert everything and just swap over, this shouldn't be an obstacle. This is a fully balanced diet, though not one for vegetarians and some people may be put off by the quantity of red meat recommended. However, the well-illustrated recipes are excellent, even inspiring.

NEW DIET REVOLUTION: DR ROBERT C. ATKINS

Robert Atkins' original *Diet Revolution* was the pioneering high-protein diet, which has now been modified and adapted. The introductory phase is still close to a classic early high-protein diet. You are permitted to eat some carbs but only 20g a day in the form of salad leaves or green vegetables. You are not allowed to eat fruit, bread, pasta, grains, starchy vegetables and the only dairy products permitted are cheese, cream and butter. Pulses, nuts and seeds are not included either. This 14-day introductory phase should be accompanied with vitamin and mineral supplements and it is important to drink enough water. You monitor your state of ketosis using a urine stick (see page 14).

In the next phase, ongoing weight loss, you increase your carbs by 5g net carbs a day until you either begin to put weight on, or stop showing signs of ketosis. (Net carbs is generally total carbs in grams minus fibre count in grams.) By that point, most dieters are consuming 40-60g net carbs a day. There are two more phases: a pre-maintenance phase you start when you are close to target, and the maintenance diet.

Sample menus, introductory phase:
Breakfast
Smoked salmon and cream cheese wraps with two hard-boiled eggs; crustless quiche with two tomato slices; or 110g cottage cheese with cinnamon and linseeds plus two crispbreads.
Lunch
Vegetable broth with white radish and prawn salad over greens; ham, spinach and cheese omelette with green salad; or homemade chicken soup.

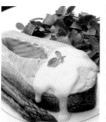

Dinner
Poached salmon with Béarnaise sauce, sautéed asparagus and a green salad; grilled steak with oven-fried turnips and a rocket and lettuce salad; or Cajun pork chops with sautéed kale and garlic.

Snacks
30g Swiss cheese; 10-20 olives; or a low-carb strawberry shake.

Ongoing weight-loss phase:
Enjoy all fish, all poultry, shellfish, meat (but watch processed products), eggs, mature cheese, salad leaves.

Reintroduce, in order:
- more salad and approved vegetables
- fresh cheese (such as ricotta)
- seeds and nuts
- berries
- wine and spirits that are low in carbs
- other fruit
- starchy vegetables
- wholegrains.

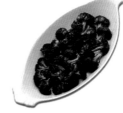

Effectiveness

Many dietitians have reservations about the extreme nature of some of the requirements of the Atkins Diet, and the content of the diet itself. If you do opt for this, then don't do the introductory phase for longer than a fortnight; do follow the recommendations – such as taking supplements and drinking lots of water – carefully. The quantity of animal fats involved is still high enough to cause concern, and the diet recommends the use of artificial sweeteners, about which many scientists have reservations. Some of the menu suggestions in *Atkins for Life* involve ingredients which may be hard to find, and the diet would be almost impossible for vegetarians and vegans to follow. Having said that, there have been many reports of successful weight loss without noticeable side-effects. If you followed it exactly, you would undoubtedly lose weight.

THE NEW HIGH-PROTEIN DIET: DR CHARLES CLARK

Charles Clark is an authority on diabetes and a professor at Griffith University in Queensland, Australia, who works both in Australia and in the UK. Spending over 20 years in the clinical management of diabetes inspired his interest in diet and nutrition, and led to him developing this diet.

The New High-Protein Diet is a straightforward high-protein diet which allows some carbs – between 40 and 60g a day – in its introductory, weight-loss phase. Clark also points out that while dietary fats do not necessarily cause weight gain, and therefore do not need to be avoided, it is important to eat 'good' fats. He draws attention to potential problems, and stresses the importance of not staying on the introductory phase for too long.

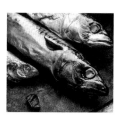 Everything containing refined carbs or processed sugars is excluded – no pasta, rice, cakes or biscuits – but you can, indeed, *must* eat a slice of wholemeal bread a day. The excluded foods can be eaten in moderation at a later stage, but not while you're trying to lose weight – and they can be avoided temporarily later on if you regain weight. Clark stresses the need to lose weight gradually, and regards the presence of ketones as an indication that you are cutting back on carbs too much. Fruits are restricted in the weight-loss phase, except for an orange a day; you can replace the orange with a vitamin C tablet and another fruit if you wish.

Foods to avoid	Restricted foods	Foods to eat without restriction
Pasta	Bread, wholemeal – one slice a day	All fresh protein from an animal source (meat, fish, shellfish)
Rice		
Flour	Milk – a very little, substitute with lemon or cream	
Potatoes and other starchy vegetables	Fruits – an orange a day in the introductory phase (or a vitamin C tablet and one other piece of fruit). Reintroduce fruit as quickly as possible once weight loss is steady	'Pure' fats – olive oil, particularly, but also butter
Refined sugar		Eggs and cheese
Breakfast cereals		Fresh non-starchy vegetables
Yoghurt		Onions and garlic, herbs and spices
Beer		Tea
Caffeinated coffee		Low-calorie soft drinks, except those high in caffeine
Fruit juice	Pulses – reintroduce when satisfied with your weight	Artificial sweeteners
Dried fruit		

Golden rules

· Eat no more than 40-60g of carbs a day.
· Restrict fruit in the weight-loss phase; no fruit juices.
· Cut out virtually all milk; the sugar in milk is often overlooked (cheese and cream are unrestricted).
· No pulses or grains at all in the weight-loss phase, except for the maximum single slice of bread a day.
· Stick to low-calorie soft drinks.
· Avoid sweet foods.
· Cut out beer and drink tea, not coffee; caffeine stimulates insulin production. Alcohol other than beer isn't prohibited but moderation is advised.
· Drink plenty of water.
· Eat as much protein as you like.
· Eat as many fresh, non-starchy vegetables as you like.
· Use 'good' fats.
· An egg a day is fine.
· 'You can't have many lapses or it won't work'.

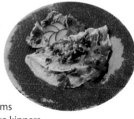

Sample menus
Breakfast

Fried bacon, mushrooms and tomato; one or two kippers with plum tomatoes; or two scrambled eggs with Parma ham and a slice of buttered toast.

Lunch

Chicken drumsticks, tomato and avocado salad; an open tomato, Mozzarella and avocado salad sandwich; or an omelette with filling.

Dinner

Lamb skewers with cucumber raita; sliced beef in oyster sauce with stir-fried vegetables; or swordfish steaks with lemon and garlic.

Effectiveness

This diet is clear and exceptionally easy to follow. You are retraining your body not to need some foods and, if you are careful, there is no reason why it shouldn't be successful. Taking a vitamin C supplement is recommended in the weight-loss phase, but this diet isn't as extreme as traditional high-protein diets. The recipes are appetising and there are sensible suggestions for exercises.

It would not be suitable for vegetarians or anyone who needs a very structured diet; it really is down to you to come up with meal plans but the guidelines are simple. It may be difficult to resist temptation, however, if you are the only person in a family following it – and giving into temptation will break the diet because what it essentially aims to do is break bad habits (or even addictions, to substances like sugar). The success of this diet depends, more than most, on your willpower as it could be easy to overdo the 'unrestricted' foods.

THE SOUTH BEACH DIET: DR ARTHUR AGATSTON

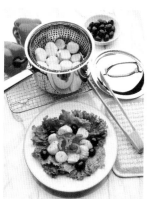

Florida cardio-logist Arthur Agatston became frustrated by the shortcomings of the diets recommended for his heart patients, particularly the low-fat, high-carb one produced by the American Heart Association. None of them seemed to work, especially over the longer term, but his patients desperately needed to lose weight. He developed his own diet, eventually published it as a book, and it soon became successful. One reason why it did so is that there is no counting, no weighing and measuring. There are clear and simple guidelines to

THE SOUTH BEACH DIET

Phase 1: Foods to enjoy	Foods to avoid
Lean cuts of beef	Fatty cuts of beef
Skinless white poultry	Chicken legs, duck, goose
Fish and shellfish	Full-fat cheeses, brie and Edam
Fat-free or low-fat cheeses	Carrots, corn, potatoes
Pistachios, peanuts, pecans	Fruit and fruit juices
Egg whites, tofu	Breads, rice, pasta
Most non-starchy vegetables	Yoghurt, milk
Olive oil	Alcohol

Phase 2: Foods to enjoy	Foods to avoid (or eat rarely)
Most fruits	White rice
Low-fat yoghurt, skimmed milk	Baked potatoes
High-fibre cereals, oatmeal	White breads
Brown rice	Biscuits
Wholewheat pasta	Carrots, corn
Popcorn	Bananas, pineapple
Red wine	Fruit juices
Multigrain bread	Watermelon
Barley	Honey/jam

Phase 3

A healthy diet following the South Beach rules and compensating for any occasional slip-ups!

follow in each of the three phases of the diet, and you're allowed to eat as much as you want – provided you stick to the guidelines.

Sample menu, Phase One

Phase one lasts for one or two weeks only and should not be followed long term. You eat lean protein and tofu, non-starchy vegetables, fat-free or low-fat cheeses, nuts and seeds, and use 'good' fats. No starchy carbs, alcohol, milk or fruit are allowed.

Breakfast
Tomato juice, an egg, two slices of bacon.
Lunch
Chopped vegetable salad with tuna, followed by sugar-free jelly for dessert.
Dinner
Baked chicken breast, roast aubergine and peppers, tossed salad with vinaigrette, followed by mocha ricotta cream.
Snacks (two a day)
Turkey roll-up with coriander mayo; celery stuffed with low-fat soft cheese.

Sample menu, Phase Two

Gradually reintroduce healthy carbs – fruit, wholegrain bread, brown rice, wholemeal pasta together with yoghurt and milk, and stay on this phase until you reach your target. Alcohol, particularly a glass of red wine, can be reintroduced in moderation during this phase. Some fruits, like bananas, are still out, as are white breads and flour, biscuits, cakes, honey and jam. If you slip up and put on weight again, return to Phase One until you get back to your ideal size.

Breakfast
Berry smoothie made with 225g yoghurt, 85g berries and crushed ice blended until smooth.
Lunch
Lemon couscous chicken, with a tomato and cucumber salad.
Dinner
Marinated rump steak, French beans with red pepper sauté, mashed cauliflower; melon.
Snacks
Fat-free yoghurt, hummus with raw vegetables.

Phase Three
The maintenance phase is the most liberal stage, and is a lifestyle rather than a diet. There are some menu ideas but the

choice is essentially yours. If you put weight back on you return to Phase One until you've lost the excess, then go back to Phase Three.

Agatston recommends judging your size from the fit of your clothes rather than weighing yourself regularly. Exercise is also recommended, and he is restrained about the need for supplements: the only one he really advises you take is fish oil.

Effectiveness

The *South Beach Diet* is an all-round healthy diet which should do no harm whatsoever to your health. It should also be easy for most people to follow: there are exact plans for those who want structure, but the principles are clear enough for the independent-minded to follow and, once out of the introductory phase, it should be possible to eat out occasionally without blowing your diet.

It is one of the few new high-protein diets to make use of carbs' glycaemic index (GI) and it resembles the GI diets in not requiring dieters to count, weigh and measure. If you are happy with that sort of freedom, then this diet may well suit you. It could, however, be possible to overeat the permitted foods and it would be difficult for vegetarians to follow.

THE VEGETARIAN LOW-CARB DIET: ROSE ELLIOT

Rose Elliot is familiar to all vegetarians as one of the foremost vegetarian cookery writers of the last 20 years. She is well known for providing excellent recipes that counter the popular impression of vegetarian food as being heavy, brown, dull and worthy. She prepared this diet with the express purpose of addressing the fact that vegetarians and vegans find many popular diets impossible to follow.

Elliot believes that most vegetarians have a tendency to eat carbs at the expense of protein, and while the *Vegetarian Low-Carb Diet* isn't strictly a very high-protein diet – it recommends about 60-80g protein per day – it could well be high in protein by most vegetarians' standards. Inspired originally by Atkins, it

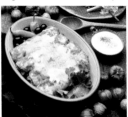

is divided into three phases. Phase One is called the Carb Cleanse; you only eat 20-30g of carbs per day and go into ketosis. This is recommended to last a fortnight. Phase Two

is called Continuing Weight Loss and you gradually increase carb levels at first, giving you a weight loss of a maximum of a kilo a week. This phase lasts until you reach target. The third phase is maintenance.
There are three basic steps: cut carbs, add fat 'to make up for lost calories' and boost protein.

This last point can be problematic for vegetarians. Meat and fish contain no carbs but all vegetarian proteins do – and those carbs have to be allowed for in the calculations. Elliot uses some proteins which will be unfamiliar to non-vegetarians, and possibly some vegetarians as well, like seitan and protein powder (soya protein isolate, whey or rice protein). Eggs are also used frequently, which would not suit vegans but there are substitutions.

Golden Rules
· Count the carbs and watch out for hidden carbs.
· Read labels.
· Eat regular meals and don't go more than six hours without eating.
· Get enough protein.
· Use 'good' fats.
· Take vitamins.
· Avoid aspartame (an artificial sweetener) and caffeine.
· Don't drink alcohol but do drink plenty of water.

Sample menus for Carb Cleanse:
Breakfast
Three-egg omelette with mushrooms and half a tomato.
Lunch
Caesar salad.
Dinner
Spinach and cream cheese gratin, with half a tomato and watercress.
Snack
100g plain Greek yoghurt with two tablespoons of ground golden flax seeds (linseeds).

Sample menus for later phases:
Breakfast
Scrambled eggs on a large mushroom; oven-baked vegan mushroom frittata; or cream cheese 'pancakes'.
Lunch
Soft goat's cheese salad with pecan nuts; aubergine and tahini dip with vegetables; or eggs Florentine.
Dinner
Smoked tofu kebabs with peanut sauce; Chinese vegetable stir-fry with ginger and garlic; or Thai coconut curry.

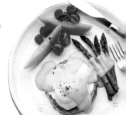

Effectiveness

The recipes are clear and easy to follow and there should be no problems sourcing most of the special ingredients in a good health-food shop. If the rest of the family is not vegetarian then it could be problematic but you're probably used to making different things for different people. The Carb Cleanse phase is quite difficult to follow without using the meal plans, though there are suggestions for how this could be done. In the second phase, carbs are reintroduced in a structured way and improvisation away from that could undermine your efforts unless you are very careful.

Following this diet carefully should bring about steady weight loss but you are advised to take a good multivitamin plus mineral supplement and drink plenty of water. It would not be advisable to follow the Carb Cleanse phase for longer than a fortnight.

THE ZONE DIET: BARRY SEARS

Barry Sears, Ph.D, a former staff member of the Massachusetts Institute of Technology (MIT), has worked on cancer treatments and hormone responses. The aim of his diet is to keep insulin (and therefore blood sugar) levels within steady limits.

The 'Zone' itself is a specific balance of foods which control hunger and burn fat by balancing your hormonal responses. Combining proteins and carbs is one way to slow the absorption of carbs and you can use this effect if you balance your diet accordingly.

In order to simplify the process, Sears has divided food into 'blocks'. One protein block contains 7g of low-fat protein – lean meat, poultry without the skin, fish, egg whites and soya. Each block of protein has to be balanced with a 9g block of complex carbs, preferably vegetables and fruit as they supply more fibre, vitamins and minerals than breads and starches. Each protein and carb block must be accompanied by a block of fat – 1.5g of 'good' fat – to slow the absorption further. All meals and snacks are based on the 1 block protein : 1 block carb : 1 block fat ratio.

The diet allows three meals a day and two snacks, and the regular spacing of these is essential to maintain steady insulin levels. The average woman should base her meals on three blocks of protein, carb and fat; the average man on four of each. In practice this can mean having one type of protein, several different vegetables, and using the fat to cook with. Salad is useful, as ten cups of green leaves are a single carb block.

Though it sounds fiddly, there are some useful general guidelines which make it considerably easier. You don't have to follow the block method: at any one meal, the protein should be no more than will cover the palm of your hand (and no thicker than it, either) and should take up about a third of your plate. The carbs should cover the other two-thirds of the plate and the fat can be used for cooking, as a salad dressing or in the form of flaked nuts or olives sprinkled on top.

There are no phases to this diet and you don't go into ketosis. There is a version aimed at vegetarians called *The Soy Zone* and Sears is now recommending that everyone, vegetarian or not, should incorporate more soya protein in their diet.

He also stresses the importance of exercise, which will help to lower insulin, but states that walking for 30 minutes a day is adequate as most insulin regulation comes from the diet. He recommends taking a daily cod liver oil supplement.

Sample menus:
Breakfast
Spicy ham omelette; blueberry cottage cheese; or yoghurt-topped apple.
Lunch
Spiced pepper steak; seafood chowder; or Mediterranean chicken salad with artichoke hearts.
Dinner
Stir-fried pork with tarragon mustard sauce; spiced lamb with spring vegetables; or a tofu and aubergine gumbo.
Dessert
Peaches with apple and almond topping; glazed spiced apple; or a raspberry-lime smoothie.

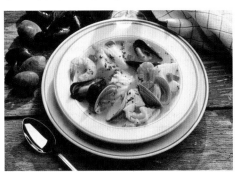

Snacks
Low-fat yoghurt and nuts;
cheese and grapes – and
even 120ml wine with 30g
cheese.

Effectiveness
The *Zone Diet* is a
healthy long-term diet
and, if followed properly –

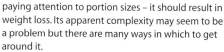

paying attention to portion sizes – it should result in
weight loss. Its apparent complexity may seem to be
a problem but there are many ways in which to get
around it.

There should be no problems with hunger. The Zone
Diet favours 'good' fats and includes enough carbs to
avoid ketosis and any of the health problems which
can be associated with it. Increasing quantities once
you have reached your target weight should prevent
further unwanted weight loss.

On the downside, if you decide to follow the strictest
calculation method of monitoring your food you are
in for a lot of weighing, measuring and adding up; on
the upside, the shortcuts should work perfectly well
providing you stick to the portion guidelines.

HOW TO USE THIS BOOK

The foods in this book are grouped into categories – Bakery, Biscuits, Condiments and Sauces, etc. – which are listed in alphabetical order in the left-hand column of each page, together with portion sizes and cooking methods, where applicable. There are some well-known branded foods but the emphasis is on whole foods, since these are the mainstay of all the high-protein, carb-controlled diets.

The portion sizes given are 'average' ones that you might eat in a single serving, such as one medium apple or 100g of chicken breast. We have also used cup measurements where they are helpful because it's easier to visualise a cup of salad than to weigh out a specific weight of lettuce leaves, especially if you are eating in a restaurant. Note: think of a teacup-full rather than a huge mug!

The first column gives the carbohydrate content of the portion in grams; the second lists its fibre content; the third column from the left gives the calorie count, in kilocalories, and the fourth and fifth give protein and fat counts in grams. The Atkins Diet asks people to consider net carbs, which is generally total carbs minus the fibre content. They give a better indication of how quickly a food will affect your blood sugar so you can use these to assess the carbs you eat whatever diet you decide to follow. For example, a slice of wheatgerm bread has 11.9g of carbs and 1.7g of fibre so the net carbs will be 10.2g.

These portion sizes may not accord with the portion sizes your diet recommends or that you wish to eat. To find the values for a 28g piece of chicken breast (a typical *Zone Diet* serving), you would have to divide the figures given by 100 and multiply by 28.

Note that values are given for cooked products rather than raw. Pasta, rice and pulses swell up to approximately three times their weight when cooked but food packaging often gives the values for their dry weight. Therefore, 75g of boiled white rice has a carb count of 23.2g while 75g of dry uncooked white rice has a carb count of 59.9g.

Values for unbranded foods have been obtained from *The Composition of Foods* (5th edition, 1991 and 6th summary edition, 2002) and *Vegetables, Herbs and Spices* (supplement, 1991), and have been reproduced by permission of Controller of Her Majesty's Stationery Office. Asda kindly supplied additional information.

The publishers are grateful to all manufacturers who gave information on their products. If you cannot find a particular food here, you can obtain much fuller listings of nutrient counts in branded foods from *Collins Gem Calorie Counter*.

CONVERSION CHART

Metric to imperial
100 grams (g) = 3.53 ounces (oz)
1 kilogram (kg) = 2.2 pounds (lb)
100 millilitres (ml) = 3.38 fluid ounces (fl oz)
1 litre = 1.76 pints

Imperial to metric
1 ounce (oz) = 28.35 grams (g)
1 pound (lb) = 453.60 grams (g)
1 stone (st) = 6.35 kilograms (kg)
1 fluid ounce (fl oz) = 29.57 millilitres (ml)
1 pint = 0.568 litres (l)

ABBREVIATIONS USED IN THE LISTINGS

g	gram
kcal	kilocalorie
ml	millilitre
n/a	not available

PORTION SIZES AT A GLANCE

It's important to be able to judge portion sizes by eye, because modern life is too complicated to start weighing every ingredient at every meal. Here are a few guidelines that will help:

BAKERY
· A medium-cut slice of bread about twice the height and width of this book will weigh around 30g.
· A 2cm thick slice of French bread is around 33g.
· A bagel the size of a can of tuna weighs around 70g.
· A muffin that fits in a fairy cake wrapper will be around 60g.
· A slice of cake weighing 75g will be roughly 7.5cm at the widest point.

BAKING PRODUCTS
· 3tsp of baking powder, flour or cornflour is 10g.

BEANS AND PULSES
· Half a cup of cooked beans weighs about 115g.

BREAKFAST CEREALS
· 30g of flaked or puffed cereal will go halfway up a normal bowl; 40g of All Bran or grapenuts will be about the same volume; and 50g of muesli or granola is half a standard bowl.

CONDIMENTS AND SAUCES
· 15ml is about a tablespoon and 5ml is a teaspoon.

DAIRY
· 15g of butter is the amount that you would spread on one slice of bread for even but not particularly thick coverage.
· A 25g piece of cheese will be around 1 x 1 x 4cm (or the size of your thumb).

FRUIT
· A medium apple or orange is about the size of a tennis ball, and weighs around 200g.
· A medium banana should fit on the average side plate, and weighs around 150g peeled.
· A half teacup of chopped fruit or berries is around 75g.

JAMS AND SPREADS
· A teaspoon of jam is about 5g and a tablespoon about 15g.
· 2 tablespoons of peanut butter, about the size of a golfball, weighs 30g.

MEAT AND POULTRY
· A 75g piece of meat or chicken would be the size of a pack of pocket tissues; a 100g piece would be more like the size of a pack of cards.

- Burgers range in size from 85g for skinny ones up to 125g for thick ones. A 'quarterpounder' is 120g.

RICE
- 2 tablespoons of dry rice will give around 75g cooked – a mound that's roughly the size of a woman's fist.

SNACKS
- 25g of nuts is roughly the amount a small child could hold in one hand.
- 25g of crisps is a large handful for an adult. The standard size for a bag of crisps is 34.5g.

VEGETABLES
- A teacup of salad greens is around 30g; half a cup of boiled cabbage is around 75g. Vegetable weights vary, but the portion sizes given in the listings relate to half a teacupful, unless otherwise stated.

COOKING TIPS

You should be aware that the way food is cooked can substantially affect its nutritional values.
- Sugar added during cooking will increase the carbohydrate content. 100g of apples stewed without sugar have just 8.1g carb, while 100g stewed with sugar have more than double the amount, at 19.1g carb.

- When you stir-fry, use a thin film of olive oil, keep stirring to prevent sticking and make sure your food is cooked evenly.

- Meats can be fried, braised, baked or grilled – but don't add any breadcrumbs or batter.

- If you boil vegetables, vitamins and minerals leach out into the cooking water; steaming, stir-frying or cooking briefly in a microwave retains more of them. Roasting is also good for bringing out the flavour of vegetables. Charles Clark's *New High Protein Diet* recommends stir-frying; in fact, buying a wok is one of his tips for success. Many of the other diets also have delicious stir-fry recipes.

- Soups, stews and casseroles preserve more of the nutritional value of foods, as vitamins and minerals will be retained in the broth.

- Remember that fats make you feel fuller so include enough in each meal to satisfy your appetite.

- In general, the shorter the cooking time, the more nutrients will be retained and the better chance you have of getting all the nutrition your body needs for good health.

The Listings

BAKERY

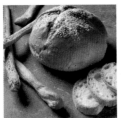

In the early days of high-protein diets, bread was completely banned – and it still is, in the introductory phase of many current high-protein diets. Wholegrain breads are often acceptable later but read labels carefully to make sure the bread really is wholegrain, not just wholemeal or multigrain, and that it doesn't contain added white flour. You need the fibre from the wholegrains. Go for stoneground bread or try pumpernickel, rye or sourdough loaves. Cakes don't belong on any weight-loss diet, and though everyone needs an occasional treat, it's best to be cautious. If you're tempted, then check labels for high levels of sugar and trans fats.

TIP: It is easier to resist the things you need to restrict if you make them difficult to get at. Freeze sliced bread rather than keeping fresh loaves in the bread bin, for example. The frozen slices can be used straight from the fridge – they toast well – but it takes thought. You can't just snack on them.

Food type	Carb (g)	Fibre (g)	Cal (kcal)	Pro (g)	Fat (g)
Bread					
Brown, 1 slice	12.6	1.5	62	2.4	0.6
Chapatis:					
made with fat, each (50g)	24.2	n/a	164	4.1	6.4
made without fat, each (50g)	21.9	n/a	101	3.7	0.5
Ciabatta, 1 slice	15.5	1.0	81	3.0	1.2
Currant loaf, 1 slice	15.3	n/a	87	2.3	2.3
French stick, 1 slice (2cm thick)	18.7	1.1	88	3.0	0.6
Garlic bread, pre-packed, frozen, 1 slice	13.6	–	110	2.4	5.5
Granary, 1 slice	14.1	1.6	71	2.9	0.7
High-bran, 1 slice	10.2	2.4	64	4.0	0.8
Malt, 1 slice	19.4	1.0	88	2.3	0.7
Naan, plain, half	31.2	1.8	177	4.9	4.5
Oatmeal, 1 slice	12.4	1.1	70	2.4	1.2
Pitta bread, white, medium:	27.7	1.2	128	4.6	0.7
white with sesame	24	1.5	131	4.8	1.8
wholewheat	20.5	3.1	114	5.4	1.2
Pitta bread, 2 mini (10g each)	11.4	0.7	52	1.7	0.3
Pumpernickel, 1 slice	14.1	1.7	68	2.3	0.5
Rye, 1 slice	13.8	n/a	66	2.5	0.5
Sourdough, 1 slice	14.7	0.9	78	2.5	0.9
Stoneground wholemeal, 1 slice	11.8	2.2	65	2.9	0.7

Food type	Carb (g)	Fibre (g)	Cal (kcal)	Pro (g)	Fat (g)
Wheatgerm, 1 slice	11.9	1.7	66	3.4	0.9
White, 1 slice	13.9	0.8	66	2.4	0.5
White, fried in oil/lard, 1 slice	14.0	0.8	149	2.4	9.7
Wholemeal, 1 slice	12.7	2.1	66	2.8	0.8
Rolls					
Bagels, each (70g):	37.2	1.5	192	7.8	1.0
onion bagels	37.7	1.5	192	7.8	1.1
sesame bagels	36.9	1.5	190	7.9	1.3
cinnamon & raisin	39.2	1.5	197	7.4	1.3
Baps, white, each (60g)	26.2	1.6	141	5.9	2.6
Brown, crusty, each (60g)	30.2	n/a	153	6.2	1.7
Brown, soft, each (60g)	26.9	2.6	142	5.9	1.9
Hamburger bun, each (60g)	29.2	n/a	158	5.4	3
White, crusty, each (60g)	32.9	1.7	157	5.5	1.3
White, soft, each (60g)	30.9	1.6	153	5.6	1.6
Wholemeal, each (60g)	27.7	3.3	147	6.3	2.0
Taco shells, each (30g)	18.4	n/a	152	2.1	7.8
Tortillas, each (30g):					
corn	18.1	n/a	103	3.0	2.1
flour	15.7	n/a	97	2.7	2.7

TIP: Some bread packaging gives nutritional information by the slice, but if it says 'per serving' it probably means 2 slices.

Food type	Carb (g)	Fibre (g)	Cal (kcal)	Pro (g)	Fat (g)
Tea Breads, Buns, Pastries					
Brioche, each (60g)	32.9	1.3	208	4.8	6.3
Chelsea bun, each (70g)	39.0	n/a	257	5.5	9.9
Croissant, each (70g)	30.3	2.2	261	5.8	13.8
Crumpet, each (50g)	15.9	1.5	91	3.0	0.4
Currant bun, each (70g)	36.8	2.0	196	5.6	3.9
Danish pastry, each (70g)	35.9	–	240	4.1	9.9
Doughnut, each (70g):					
jam	34.1	n/a	235	4.0	10.1
ring	33.1	–	282	4.3	15.7
Eccles cake, each (60g)	33.8	n/a	232	2.4	10.7
Fruit loaf, slice (70g)	44.9	n/a	217	4.9	3.4
Hot cross bun, each (70g)	40.9	n/a	218	5.2	4.9
Muffin, each (70g):					
English	29.5	2.3	160	7.1	1.5
blueberry	34.9	0.8	300	3	0.8
Potato scone, each (60g)	25.2	2.6	124	2.8	1.3
Raisin and cinnamon					
loaf, slice (70g)	35	2.2	182	4.9	2.9
Scone, each (60g):					
fruit	30.7	1.7	207	4.8	7.2

TIP: If you're desperate for a sandwich, or in a situation where sandwiches are the only choice, then choose a diet-friendly filling and remove the top slice of bread, turning it into an open sandwich.

Food type	Carb (g)	Fibre (g)	Cal (kcal)	Pro (g)	Fat (g)
Scones contd:					
plain	32.2	n/a	218	4.3	8.9
wholemeal	25.9	n/a	197	5.3	8.8
Scotch pancake, each (60g)	29.8	0.7	158	4.0	2.7
Cakes and Cream Cakes					
Almond slice (50g bar)	20.6	0.8	212	6.5	12.9
Apple Danish (50g bar)	20.7	1.1	165	3.3	7.8
Bakewell slice (50g)	19.4	0.4	150	1.5	7.4
Banana cake, slice (75g)	41.9	0.5	260	2.4	6
Battenburg, slice (75g)	52.7	1.0	323	5.2	10.1
Brownies, chocolate, each (75g)	40.6	1.6	365	3.8	20.7
Caramel shortcake, piece (50g)	27.6	0.5	248	2	14.5
Carrot cake, slice (75g)	44.9	0.9	300	2.4	12.3
Chocolate cake, slice (75g)	42.3	1	268	4.3	10.5
Chocolate mini roll, each (50g)	27.4	0.7	222	2.2	11.1
Chocolate sandwich sponge, slice (50g)	24.0	0.9	192	2.0	9.8
Date and walnut loaf, slice (75g)	30.8	0.8	264	4.4	13.7

TIP: Many 'wholemeal' and rye breads still use highly refined flour which can cause bloating and blood sugar peaks.

Food type	Carb (g)	Fibre (g)	Cal (kcal)	Pro (g)	Fat (g)
Chocolate éclair, each (75g)	19.6	n/a	297	4.2	23.0
Fancy cake, iced, each (50g)	34.5	–	178	1.9	4.6
Flapjack, oat, each (75g)	46.8	n/a	370	3.6	20.3
Fruit cake, slice (75g):					
plain	43.4	–	278	3.8	11.1
rich	44.9	n/a	257	2.9	8.5
rich, iced	49.4	–	263	2.7	7.4
wholemeal	39.3	n/a	274	4.5	12.1
Ginger cake, slice (75g)	46.4	0.9	295	2.6	11.0
Greek pastries (sweet),					
each (50g)	20	–	161	2.4	8.5
Lemon cake, slice (75g)	41.6	0.8	289	3.4	13.5
Marble cake, slice (75g)	41.6	0.9	278	3.9	10.5
Madeira cake, slice (75g)	43.8	–	283	4.1	11.3
Mince pie, each (50g)	30	0.8	198	1.9	7.8
Sponge cake, slice (50g):					
plain	26.3	n/a	234	3.2	13.6
fat-free	26.5	n/a	151	5	3.5
jam-filled	32.1	n/a	151	2.1	2.5
with butter icing	26.2	0.3	245	2.3	15.5
Swiss roll, original, slice (50g)	30.3	0.6	146	2.6	1.6
Trifle sponge, each (50g)	33.6	0.5	162	2.6	2.0

TIP: Use oatcakes instead of bread with cold meats, pâtés and cheese.
They're high-fibre, low GI and low-calorie.

BAKING PRODUCTS

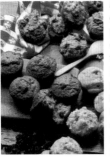

Most high-protein, low-carb diets exclude flour and pastry during their introductory phases, and restrict them thereafter. Many baking ingredients will simply give you a blood-sugar high. White flour should be avoided completely; instead go for stoneground wholemeal or rye flour, which are both higher in fibre. You can get a low-carb soya flour (see the vegetarian listings on pages 200–5) but it can be expensive, and though it's lower in carbs than normal flour it is much higher in fat – and calories. If you do bake, incorporate healthy ingredients like nuts, seeds and dried fruits, checking out local health-food shops who will often have a more interesting selection than supermarkets.

TIP: Many of the high-protein or low-carb recipe books recommend using ground almonds instead of flour. You can make your own by pulverising almonds in a blender or food processor.

Food type	Carb (g)	Fibre (g)	Cal (kcal)	Pro (g)	Fat (g)
Baking Agents					
Baking powder, 10g (3tsp)	3.8	n/a	16	0.5	–
Cornflour, 25g	22.9	n/a	88	0.1	0.2
Flour, 100g:					
rye, whole	75.9	n/a	335	8.2	2.0
wheat, brown	68.5	n/a	324	12.6	2.0
wheat, white, breadmaking	70	3.1	337	11.0	1.4
wheat, white, plain	71	3.1	336	10.0	1.3
wheat, white, self-raising	72	2.0	343	11.0	1.2
wheat, wholemeal	58.0	9	308	14.0	2.2
Ground rice, 100g	86.8	0.5	361	6.5	1
Pastry, 50g:					
filo, uncooked	31	1	156	4.5	1.5
flaky, cooked	23	n/a	282	2.8	20.5
puff, uncooked	15	0.8	210	2.5	15.5
shortcrust, cooked	27.2	n/a	262	3.3	16.3
shortcrust, mix	30.4	1.2	234	3.7	11.6
wholemeal, cooked	22.3	n/a	251	4.5	16.6
Sugar, caster, 50g	50	–	200	–	–
Yeast, bakers'					
compressed, 25g	0.3	n/a	13	2.9	0.1
dried, 15g	0.5	n/a	25	5.3	0.2

TIP: Try to avoid buying prepared mixes and fillings; they are often very high in ingredients you should be trying to avoid.

Food type	Carb (g)	Fibre (g)	Cal (kcal)	Pro (g)	Fat (g)
Fats					
Butter, 25g	Tr	n/a	225	Tr	25
Cooking fat, 25g	–	–	225	–	25
Lard, 1tbsp	–	n/a	134	Tr	14.9
Margarine, hard (over 80% animal/vegetable fat), 25g	0.3	n/a	180	0.1	19.8
Margarine, soft (over 80% polyunsaturated fat), 25g	0.1	n/a	187	Tr	20.7
Suet, shredded, 1 tbsp	1.8	n/a	124	Tr	13
Mixes					
Batter mix, 100g	77.2	3.7	338	9.3	1.2
Cheesecake mix, 100g:					
strawberry	31.5	n/a	258	3	12
toffee	37.5	n/a	342	3.2	19.3
Crumble mix, 100g	67.6	1.5	422	5.5	16.3
Egg custard mix, no bake, 100g	14.1	0.5	96	4.4	2.4
Madeira cake mix, 100g	56	n/a	339	4.9	12.4
Pancake mix, 100g	65.9	2.3	322	13.4	2.5
Victoria sponge mix, 100g	52	n/a	367	6	15

TIP: Wholemeal stoneground flour isn't always heavy – some brands are much lighter than others, so experiment if you don't like the first one you try.

Food type	Carb (g)	Fibre (g)	Cal (kcal)	Pro (g)	Fat (g)
Sundries					
Almonds, flaked/ground, 25g	1.8	1.8	158	6.3	14
Cherries, *glacé*, 25g	16.6	n/a	63	0.1	–
Cherry pie filling, 100g	21.5	n/a	82	0.4	Tr
Currants, dried, 25g	17	n/a	67	0.6	0.1
Ginger, *glacé*, 25g	18.6	n/a	76	0.1	0.2
Lemon juice, 50ml	0.8	n/a	4	0.2	Tr
Marzipan, 50g	33.8	–	195	2.7	6.4
Mincemeat (sweet), 50g	31.1	n/a	137	0.3	2.2
Mixed peel, 50g	14.8	n/a	58	0.1	0.2
Raisins, seedless, 25g	17.3	0.5	72	0.5	0.1
Royal icing, 50g	48.8	–	195	0.7	–
Sultanas, 25g	17.4	0.5	69	0.7	0.1

TIP: Remember that baked goods are excluded from the introductory phase of most high-protein diets and are generally restricted there-after. If you are baking for others, then make sure you don't join in – and 'testing' counts as joining in.

BEANS, PULSES AND CEREALS

Pulses are a good source of protein, as well as micronutrients and fibre, so incorporate them in your diet. You need to watch quantities because of their carb content, but adding some to soups and casseroles is a good idea, and they make a great base for salads. One advantage of using them is that they fill you up; their fibre content means that they are digested relatively slowly. Avoid most tinned baked beans in tomato sauce as they are often high in sugar, but a few tins of plain pulses are a good storecupboard standby – haricots and chickpeas are probably the most versatile. Dried pulses will need soaking before being cooked; they should always be rinsed and checked for any small pieces of grit.

TIP: Try a lentil and roast pepper salad. Preheat the oven to 200ºC /gas mark 6. Cut two red peppers in half, remove the seeds and put them, skin side uppermost, into a roasting tin. Cook for 35–40 minutes until they begin to blister. Peel when cool enough to handle and cut them into squares. Rinse about 200g green lentils, cover with fresh water, bring to the boil and simmer briefly until they are cooked but retain a bit of bite. Drain and put in a bowl; add the peppers, some chopped parsley, and season. Dress with olive oil and a little lemon juice, and stir gently. Serve slightly warm, or leave for the flavours to blend together.

Food type	Carb (g)	Fibre (g)	Cal (kcal)	Pro (g)	Fat (g)
Beans and Pulses					
Aduki beans, 115g	25.9	n/a	141	10.7	0.2
Baked beans, small can (200g):					
in tomato sauce	30.6	n/a	168	10.4	1.2
tomato sauce, no added sugar	22.6	7.4	132	9.4	0.4
Baked beans with pork					
sausages, small can (200g)	22.0	6.0	194	11.2	6.8
Baked beans with					
vegetable sausages,					
small can (200g)	24.4	5.8	210	12.0	7.2
Blackeyed beans, 115g	22.9	n/a	133	10.1	0.8
Borlotti beans, half can (100g)	20.5	5.5	121	8.7	0.5
Broad beans, small can (200g)	22	10	164	16	1.4
Butter beans:					
small can (200g)	27.8	9.6	166	12.0	0.8
dried, boiled (115g)	21.2	6	118	8.2	0.7
Cannellini beans,					
small can (200g)	28	12	174	14	0.6
Chick peas:					
small can (200g)	32.2	n/a	230	14.4	5.8
dried, boiled (115g)	20.9	n/a	139	9.7	2.4

TIP: Combine cooked beans with crunchy raw vegetables like red onion, chopped fennel, celery and chopped carrot for a sustaining and nutritious salad.

Food type	Carb (g)	Fibre (g)	Cal (kcal)	Pro (g)	Fat (g)
Chilli beans, small can (200g)	28	7.4	160	9.6	1
Flageolet beans, half can (100g)	22.4	2.4	132	9.0	0.7
Haricot beans, 115g					
dried, boiled	19.8	7	109	7.6	0.6
Hummus, 2 tbsp	3.3	n/a	53	2.2	3.6
Lentils, 115g:					
green/brown, boiled	19.4	n/a	121	10.1	0.8
red, split, boiled	20.1	n/a	115	8.7	0.5
Marrow fat peas:					
small can (200g)	28	9.6	168	12	0.8
quick-soak, 115g	48.2	16.1	334	29.1	2.8
Mung beans, 115g					
boiled	17.6	n/a	105	8.7	0.5
Pinto beans:					
boiled, 115g	27.5	–	158	10.2	0.8
refried, 2 tbsp	4.6	–	32	1.9	0.3
Red kidney beans:					
small can (200g)	27	12.8	182	16.2	1.0
boiled, 115g	20	n/a	118	9.7	0.6
Soya beans, 115g					
dried, boiled	5.9	n/a	162	16.1	8.4

TIP: There's no need to soak red or green lentils before cooking. Just rinse them and boil in fresh water until they are soft – which can take as little as 10 minutes if they are very fresh.

Food type	Carb (g)	Fibre (g)	Cal (kcal)	Pro (g)	Fat (g)
Split peas, 115g, *boiled*	26.1	3.1	1454	9.5	1
Tofu (soya bean curd), 2 tbsp:					
steamed	0.9	–	94	10.4	5.4
fried	2.6	–	337	30.3	22.9
Cereals					
Barley, pearl, 100g	83.6	7.3	360	7.9	1.7
Bran, 100g:					
wheat, dry	26.8	n/a	206	14.1	5.5
Bulgur wheat, dry, 100g	74	3.1	357	12	1.4
Couscous, dry, 100g	72.5	2	355	13.5	1.9
Cracked wheat, 100g	74	3.1	357	12	1.4
Polenta, ready-made, 100g	15.7	n/a	72	1.6	0.3
Wheatgerm, 100g	44.7	n/a	357	26.7	9.2
Fresh beans & peas:					
see Vegetables					
For more soya products:					
see Vegetarian					

TIP: Beans, lentils, nuts and green vegetables are good sources of folate, which seems to reduce the risk of developing breast cancer.

BISCUITS, CRACKERS AND CRISPBREADS

Sweet biscuits should be avoided, not only because they are high in sugar, fat and calories but also because they are high in trans fats, which are the ones you want to avoid (see page 20). They may also have high salt levels, so check labels very carefully before giving into temptation. Even oatcakes, recommended on several high-protein diets, can be high in trans fats. Read the packaging and opt for healthy varieties which aren't so damaging to your diet (or your health). But before you think about having a quick biscuit, it is worth remembering that it can be very difficult to stop at one.

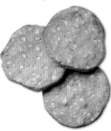

TIP: When you get the urge for a biscuit, try a few nuts instead. They are much better for you and won't break your diet – as long as you don't eat lots. Limit yourself to 15 almonds or 30 pistachios.

Food type	Carb (g)	Fibre (g)	Cal (kcal)	Pro (g)	Fat (g)
Sweet Biscuits					
Bourbon creams, each	7	n/a	47	n/a	1.9
Caramel wafers, each	6.7	n/a	45	0.5	2
Chocolate chip cookies, each	5.7	n/a	43	0.6	2
Chocolate cream wafers, each	3.2	n/a	26	0.3	1.4
Chocolate fingers, each:					
milk & plain chocolate	6.3	n/a	52	0.7	2.7
white chocolate	6.1	n/a	53	0.6	3
Shortcake cream sandwich					
fruit	9.2	0.3	75	0.9	3.8
milk chocolate	9.4	0.3	77	0.9	3.9
mint	9.4	0.3	78	0.8	4
orange	9.3	0.3	78	0.8	4.1
Custard creams, each	6.9	0.2	51	0.6	2.3
Digestive biscuits, each:					
uncoated	8.6	–	58	0.8	2.5
chocolate (milk & plain)	10	–	74	1	3.6
Fig rolls each	6.8	0.5	36	0.4	0.8
Garibaldi (plain), each	7.1	0.3	40	0.5	1.0
Gingernuts, each	8	–	44	0.6	1.3
Gipsy creams, each	9.9	0.4	77	0.7	3.8
Jaffa cakes, each	7.0	0.2	37	0.5	0.8
Lemon puff, each	6.2	0.2	52	0.7	2.7
Nice biscuits, each	6.9	0.2	49	0.7	2.1
Oat & raisin biscuits, each	6.3	0.4	47	0.8	2.1

Food type	Carb (g)	Fibre (g)	Cal (kcal)	Pro (g)	Fat (g)
Rich tea biscuits, each	7.2	0.3	46	0.7	1.6
Shortbread fingers, each	12.8	0.4	100	1.2	5.2
Shortcake biscuits, each	6.5	n/a	49	0.6	2.3
Stem ginger cookies, diet, each	6.5	0.1	40	0.5	1.3
Viennese whirls, each	2.3	0.1	21	0.2	1.3
Wafer biscuits, cream-filled, each	4.6	–	37	0.3	2.1
Crackers and Crispbreads					
Bran crackers, 4	12.6	0.6	91	1.9	3.6
Cheese crackers , 4	8.3	0.4	81	1.5	4.7
Cornish wafers, each	5.4	0.2	53	0.8	3.1
Crackerbread, each:					
original	7.6	0.3	38	1	0.3
cheese-flavoured	7.5	0.3	38	1.3	0.3
high-fibre	6.2	1.6	32	1.3	0.3
Crackers, salted, 5:					
cheese	8.4	0.3	74	1.6	3.8
original	8.3	0.3	76	1	4.3
Cream crackers, each	5.7	0.3	36	0.8	1.1
Matzo crackers, each	8.5	0.3	37	1	0.2
Oatcakes, each:					
cheese	5.4	0.6	47	1.3	2.5

TIP: Have a bran oatcake spread with cream cheese rather than a sweet biscuit, for a high-fibre snack.

Food type	Carb (g)	Fibre (g)	Cal (kcal)	Pro (g)	Fat (g)
Oatcakes, *contd*:					
fine	6.3	0.9	46	1	2.2
organic	7.1	0.9	42	0.9	1.6
rough	6.4	0.8	43	1.2	1.8
traditional	5.8	0.8	43	1.1	1.7
Rye crispbread, each:					
dark rye	6.5	1.8	31	0.9	0.1
multigrain	5.7	1.7	33	1.1	0.6
original	6.7	1.7	33	1.1	0.1
sesame	6	1.6	34	0.9	0.6
Water biscuits, 3:					
high bake	7.6	0.3	41	1	0.7
regular (table)	7.5	0.4	41	1	0.8
Wholemeal crackers, 4	10.8	0.7	62	1.5	1.7

See also Snacks and dips

TIP: If you know you can't control yourself with a particular food then it may be best to avoid it. Cheese biscuits are particularly tempting; one is never enough and before you know it you've eaten half the packet.

BREAKFAST CEREALS AND CEREAL BARS

Cereals are banned in the introductory phases of most high-protein diets, and breakfast can pose a problem for some dieters, but it doesn't have to be bacon and eggs every day – and it's much better if it isn't. Once past the initial phase most diets permit wholegrain breakfast cereals, whole-oat (not instant) porridge and muesli as long as they have no added sugar. Don't be tempted to miss out on breakfast, though; it's essential for success and helps keep blood-sugar levels on an even keel. Cereal bars present problems to the high-protein dieter and should really be avoided; if you need something quick and easy then go for an almost-instant smoothie by blending natural yoghurt and frozen berries together.

TIP: If you really like the taste of orange in the mornings, then have the whole fruit instead of the juice.

Food type	Carb (g)	Fibre (g)	Cal (kcal)	Pro (g)	Fat (g)
Breakfast Cereals					
Bran flakes, 30g	19.8	4.5	97	3	0.6
Cheerios, 40g:	30.1	2.6	148	3.2	1.6
honey-nut	31.3	2.1	150	2.8	1.5
Cornflakes, 30g:	23.4	0.9	112	2.1	0.3
Crunchy nut	24.9	0.8	118	1.8	1.2
Sugar coated	26.1	0.6	111	1.4	0.2
Chocolate sugar coated	24.0	1.1	118	1.5	1.8
Fruit 'n' Fibre, 30g	20.4	2.7	107	2.4	1.8
Grape Nuts, 40g	29	3.4	138	4.2	0.8
High Fibre Bran, 40g	18.4	10.8	112	5.6	1.8
Low fat flakes, 30g:	22.5	0.8	112	4.8	0.3
with red berries	22.8	0.9	111	4.2	0.3
Malted Wheats, 30g	21.9	2.8	108	3.2	0.8
Multi-grain cereal, 30g	24	1.5	113	2.4	0.8
Oat Bran Flakes, 30g	20.1	0.6	99	3	0.6
Oat Krunchies, 30g	18.9	3.3	108	3.2	2.1
Puffed Rice, 30g:	26.1	0.3	114	1.8	0.3
chocolate	25.2	0.6	115	1.5	0.9
sugar coated	27	0.3	115	1.4	0.2
Puffed Wheat, 30g	18.7	1.7	98	4.6	0.4

TIP: The most successful dieters – the ones who get to their target and then maintain their new weight – are those who eat breakfast, so don't be tempted to go without.

Food type	Carb (g)	Fibre (g)	Cal (kcal)	Pro (g)	Fat (g)
Shredded wheat bisks, 30g:	20.3	3.5	102	3.5	0.8
bite-size	21.0	3.6	105	3.5	0.8
sugar coated	21.6	2.7	105	3	0.6
fruit-filled	20.6	2.7	106	2.5	1.5
honey nut	20.6	2.8	113	3.4	2
Sultana Bran, 30g	20.1	0.4	95	2.4	0.6
Wheat bisks , 30g	20.4	3.0	101	3.5	0.6
Hot Cereals					
Instant Porridge					
baked apple	71	5.5	374	8	6
berry burst	71	5.5	374	8	6
golden syrup	71	6	372	7.5	6
Oatbran, 100g	49.7	15.2	345	14.8	9.7
Oatmeal, medium or fine, 100g	60.4	8.5	359	11	8.1
Oats, 100g:					
instant	60.4	8.5	359	11	8.1
jumbo	60.4	8.5	359	11	8.1
organic	61.5	8.0	363	12.5	7.4
rolled	62	7	368	11	8

TIP: The hot cereal measurement of 100g given above includes the water needed to cook it. If you use milk instead of water, then you'll need to consider the extra calories – and carbs. On pages 105–6 you'll find nutritional information on different kinds of milk.

Food type	Carb (g)	Fibre (g)	Cal (kcal)	Pro (g)	Fat (g)
Porridge (cooked), 100g:					
made with water	8.1	n/a	46	1.4	1.1
made with whole milk	12.6	n/a	113	4.8	5.1
Muesli					
Crunchy Oat Cereal, 50g:					
maple & pecan	30.0	3.3	224	5	9.4
raisin & almond	33	2.8	211	3.5	7.2
sultana & apple	29.6	6.2	189	3.8	6.1
Muesli, 50g:	33	3.8	182	5	3.4
apricot	29.5	2.8	142	3.9	1.8
deluxe	28.1	5.8	172	5.4	5
high fibre	35.4	3	158	5.2	3
natural	31.5	4.3	173	4.8	3.1
organic	29.8	4.5	177	4.5	4.4
swiss-style	36.1	n/a	182	4.9	3
swiss-style, organic	31.5	3.7	180	4.9	3.8
with no added sugar	33.6	n/a	183	5.3	3.9

TIP: Cook a high-protein breakfast in a healthy way. Have the egg boiled or poached, and grill the bacon in a pan with a drip tray. Alternatively, dry fry the egg with the bacon and don't add any extra fat. Choose back bacon rather than streaky and trim the rind – there will still be plenty of fat to cook it in. Blot it on kitchen paper once it's cooked, before putting it on your plate.

Food type	Carb (g)	Fibre (g)	Cal (kcal)	Pro (g)	Fat (g)
Cereal Bars					
Apple & blackberry, 30g	20.8	1.5	117	1.6	3.1
Banana, 30g	27.6	2	152	2.3	2
Cornflakes & milk bar, 30g	19.8	0.6	132	2.7	4.8
Fruit & Nut Break, 30g	23.7	2	170	3.0	7.0
Fruit and oats crisp, 30g:					
Apricot	21.3	2.1	122	1.7	3.3
Raisin & Hazelnut	20.4	1.3	142	2.1	5.8
Low fat flakes & milk bar, 30g	20.7	0.4	135	2.1	4.8
Muesli bar, 30g	30.6	2	178	2.7	5
Multi-grain bar, 30g:					
Apple	19.8	1.1	106	1.2	2.7
Cappuccino	19.8	0.7	111	1.4	3
Cherry	20.1	1.2	104	1.2	2.4
Chocolate	19.8	1.2	110	1.4	3.0
Orange	19.5	1.2	105	1.2	2.7
Strawberry	20.1	1.1	107	1.2	2.7
Oat and wheat bar, 30g:	22.5	0.6	117	2.1	2.1
Chocolate chip	17.7	0.5	147	2.1	7.2
Roasted nut	16.4	0.4	151	2.7	8
Puffed rice & milk bar, 30g	20.4	0.1	124	2.1	3.9

TIP: Be wary of cereal bars; they often contain lots of sugar and other ingredients you are advised to avoid on high-protein diets. Read the packaging carefully. If you can't resist, go for a high-fibre muesli bar.

Food type	Carb (g)	Fibre (g)	Cal (kcal)	Pro (g)	Fat (g)
Strawberry & yoghurt, 30g	21.0	1.1	119	1.7	3.1
Sugar coated flakes & milk bar, 30g	20.7	0.5	114	2.4	4.5

TIP: Keep a food diary. It will help you to become aware of the times when you are most tempted to snack, whether mid-afternoon or at certain times of the month. Forewarned is forearmed!

CONDIMENTS, SAUCES AND GRAVY

Most prepared sauces, chutneys, ketchups and pickles are too high in sugar and flour to be part of any high-protein diet but sauces are a good way of adding extra taste to your food. The answer is to make your own, avoiding any ingredients which are off-limits – you'll find easy recipes in most high-protein diet books. Think about other ways of adding flavour, too: tabasco, fresh chopped chillis, ginger, lemongrass and soy are all great with 'oriental' dishes, and natural yoghurt can make a good accompaniment, especially to Indian or Middle Eastern food. The use of herbs, spices and garlic helps almost any savoury dish, and cinnamon is lovely with cooked pears or stewed apple.

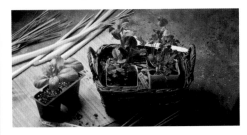

TIP: The simplest way of reducing your salt intake is to avoid processed foods and ready meals.

Food type	Carb (g)	Fibre (g)	Cal (kcal)	Pro (g)	Fat (g)
Table Sauces					
Apple sauce, 1 tbsp	4	0.2	16	–	Tr
Barbecue sauce, 1 tbsp	4.1	0.1	18	0.1	–
Beetroot in redcurrant jelly 1 tbsp	6.1	n/a	25	0.1	Tr
Brown fruity sauce, 1 tbsp	3.6	0.2	17	0.1	–
Brown sauce, 1 tbsp	3.4	n/a	15	0.2	–
Burger sauce, 1 tbsp	1.8	Tr	36	0.2	3.1
Chilli sauce, 1 tsp	1.7	–	7	0.1	Tr
Cranberry jelly, 1 tbsp	10	–	40	Tr	Tr
Cranberry sauce, 1 tbsp	6.8	n/a	27	–	–
Garlic sauce, 1 tsp	0.9	n/a	17	0.1	1.5
Ginger sauce, 1 tsp	1.4	–	6	–	–
Horseradish, creamed, 2 tsp	2	0.2	18	0.2	1
Horseradish relish, 2 tsp	1	0.3	11	0.2	0.6
Horseradish sauce, 2 tsp	1.8	n/a	15	0.2	0.8
Mint jelly, 1 tbsp	10	n/a	40	Tr	–
Mint sauce, 1 tbsp	1.9	n/a	9	0.2	–
Mushroom ketchup, 1 tbsp	0.8	Tr	4	0.1	–
Redcurrant jelly, 1 tbsp	9.8	n/a	39	–	–
Soy sauce, 2 tsp	0.8	n/a	4	0.3	Tr

TIP: Chop red peppers roughly and boil them with whole cloves of garlic until they are soft. Pop the garlic cloves out of their skins and blend them together with the peppers to make a tasty purée.

Food type	Carb (g)	Fibre (g)	Cal (kcal)	Pro (g)	Fat (g)
Tabasco, 1 tsp	–	–	–	–	–
Tartare sauce, 1 tbsp	1.3	n/a	77	0.1	7.9
Tomato ketchup, 1 tbsp	4.7	n/a	19	0.3	–
Wild rowan jelly, 2 tsp	6.5	n/a	27	–	–
Worcestershire sauce, 1 tsp	1.0	–	4	–	–
Mustards					
Dijon mustard, 1 tsp	0.1	0.1	5	0.3	0.4
English mustard, 1 tsp	0.9	0.1	9	0.3	0.4
French mustard, 1 tsp	0.6	–	7	0.3	0.3
Honey mustard, 1 tsp	1.2	0.3	9	0.3	0.2
Horseradish mustard, 1 tsp	1.2	0.2	8	0.3	0.2
Peppercorn mustard, 1 tsp	0.8	0.3	7	0.4	0.3
Wholegrain mustard, 1tsp:	0.5	0.2	8	0.5	0.5
hot, 1 tsp	0.6	0.4	7	0.4	0.2
Pickles and Chutneys					
Apple chutney, 1 tbsp	7.3	n/a	28	0.1	–
Barbecue relish, 1 tbsp	3.1	n/a	14	0.3	–
Chunky fruit chutney, 1 tbsp:	3.9	n/a	16	0.1	–
small chunk	–	0.2	21	0.1	–

TIP: Japanese shoyu is less salty than both light and dark soy sauce, and dark soy is sweeter. Use light soy during cooking, as dark soy can be overwhelming.

Food type	Carb (g)	Fibre (g)	Cal (kcal)	Pro (g)	Fat (g)
Chunky fruit chutney, *contd:*					
spicy	5.1	0.2	21	0.1	–
Lime pickle, 1 tbsp	0.6	0.1	29	0.3	2.8
Mango chutney, 1 tbsp	7.5	0.2	31	0.1	–
Mango with ginger chutney					
1 tbsp	6.9	0.1	28	0.1	–
Mediterranean chutney, 1 tbsp	3.9	0.2	17.9	0.3	0.1
Mustard pickle, mild, 1 tbsp	3.8	0.1	19	0.3	0.2
Piccalilli, 1 tbsp	3.2	0.1	16	0.2	0.1
Ploughman's pickle, 1 tbsp	4	0.1	17	0.1	–
Sandwich pickle, tangy, 1 tbsp	4.7	0.1	20	0.1	–
Sauerkraut, 2 tbsp	0.4	n/a	3	0.4	Tr
Spiced fruit chutney, 1 tbsp	5.1	n/a	21	0.1	–
Spreadable chutney, 1 tbsp	8.8	0.2	36	–	–
Sweet chilli dipping sauce,					
1 tbsp	7.8	0.1	33	0.1	–
Sweet pickle, 1 tbsp	5.4	n/a	21	0.1	–
Tomato chutney, 1 tbsp	4.6	n/a	19	0.2	–
Tomato pickle, tangy, 1 tbsp	5.2	0.4	25	0.5	–
Tomato with red pepper					
chutney, 1 tbsp	5.7	0.2	25	0.3	

TIP: Fresh ginger is a great addition to stir-fries. It goes mouldy quite quickly so peel it and store it in the freezer in a plastic bag; it can then be grated from frozen.

Food type	Carb (g)	Fibre (g)	Cal (kcal)	Pro (g)	Fat (g)
Salad Dressings					
Balsamic dressing, 2 tbsp	2.2	–	92	0.1	9.1
Blue cheese dressing, 2 tbsp	2.6	n/a	137	0.6	13.9
Blue cheese-flavoured low-fat dressing, 2 tbsp	1.8	–	18	0.5	1
Creamy Caesar dressing, 2 tbsp	2.4	–	101	0.9	9.6
Caesar-style low-fat dressing, 2 tbsp	4.4	0.1	24	1	0.3
Creamy low-fat salad dressing, 2 tbsp	4.5	n/a	37	0.2	2
French dressing, 2 tbsp	1.4	–	139	–	14.9
Italian dressing, 2 tbsp	1.7	0.1	36	–	3.1
fat free	2	0.2	10	–	Tr
Mayonnaise, 1 tbsp	0.3	–	109	0.2	11.9
light, reduced calorie, 1 tbsp	2.5	0.2	96	0.3	9.5
Salad cream, 1 tbsp	2.5	–	52	0.2	4.7
light, 1 tbsp	2	Tr	36	0.3	3
Seafood sauce, 1 tbsp	1.5	0.1	80	0.3	8.1
Thousand Island, 1 tbsp	2.9	0.1	55	0.1	4.7
fat free, 1 tbsp	3	0.4	13	0.1	–
Vinaigrette, 2 tbsp	1.4	–	139	–	14.8

TIP: For a very low-calorie mayonnaise, mix mayo with the same quantity of low-fat yoghurt. Don't forget that shop-bought low-cal mayo may be higher in carbs than the standard variety – check labels.

Food type	Carb (g)	Fibre (g)	Cal (kcal)	Pro (g)	Fat (g)
Vinegars					
Balsamic vinegar, 1 tbsp	3.2	–	15	Tr	–
Cider vinegar, 1 tbsp	0.2	–	3	–	–
Red wine vinegar, 1 tbsp	0.1	–	4	–	–
Sherry vinegar, 1 tbsp	0.3	–	4	0.1	–
White wine vinegar, 1 tbsp	0.1	–	3	–	–
Cooking Sauces					
Bread sauce, 100ml:					
made with semi-skimmed milk	15.3	n/a	97	4.2	2.5
made with whole milk	15.2	n/a	110	4.1	4
Cheese sauce, 100ml:					
made with semi-skimmed milk	8.8	n/a	181	8.2	12.8
made with whole milk	8.7	n/a	198	8.1	14.8
Curry sauce, canned, 100ml	7.1	n/a	78	1.5	5
Onion sauce, 100ml:					
made with semi-skimmed milk	8.2	n/a	88	3	5.1
made with whole milk	8.1	n/a	101	2.9	6.6
Pesto:					
fresh, homemade 100ml	6	1.4	45	2.2	1.3
green pesto, jar, 100ml	0.8	1.4	374	5	39

TIP: Cook-in sauces of all kinds are often high in ingredients which are better avoided, including sugar in all its various forms. Read labels and think about how to come up with your own version.

Food type	Carb (g)	Fibre (g)	Cal (kcal)	Pro (g)	Fat (g)
Pesto *contd*:					
red pesto, jar, 100ml	3.1	0.4	358	4.1	36.6
Tomato & basil, fresh, 100ml	8.8	1.3	51	1.8	0.9
White sauce, 100ml:					
made with semi-skimmed milk	10.7	n/a	130	4.4	8
made with whole milk	10.6	n/a	151	4.2	10.3
For more pasta sauces, *see under*: Pasta and Pizza					
Stock Cubes					
Beef, each	2.3	Tr	32	0.9	2.3
Chicken, each	2.3	Tr	32	0.9	1.8
Fish, each	0.5	Tr	32	1.8	2.3
Garlic herb & spice, each	5.3	0.4	33	1.5	0.6
Ham , each	1.8	Tr	32	1.4	1.8
Lamb, each	0.5	Tr	32	1.4	2.3
Rice saffron, each	1.4	0.4	32	1.6	2.2
Pork, each	1.4	Tr	32	1.4	2.3
Vegetable, each	1.4	Tr	45	1.4	4.1
Yeast extract, each	2.8	n/a	27	2.7	0.5

TIP: Watch out for ketchup. You don't generally use much, but it is still packed with sugar. Find alternatives, like fresh tomato slices and dill pickles with a burger, or home-flavoured mayo with fish.

Food type	Carb (g)	Fibre (g)	Cal (kcal)	Pro (g)	Fat (g)
Gravy Granules					
Gravy powder, 5g	3.1	–	13	0.1	–
Gravy instant granules, 5g	2.9	0.1	19	0.1	0.8
Swiss Vegetable					
Bouillon powder, 4g	0.7	n/a	4	0.3	–
Vegetable gravy granules, 5g	3	0.2	15	0.4	0.2

TIP: Don't choose bottled salad dressings; just stick to a drizzle of olive oil and good vinegar or lemon juice. Make a simple vinaigrette by mixing three measures of olive oil with one of balsamic vinegar in a screw-top jar and adding some Dijon mustard to taste. Put the top on firmly and shake the jar well.

DAIRY

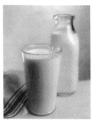

It is best to ensure that your diet includes some dairy products every day, but you need to be careful about what you choose, and how much you eat. Most cheeses, creams and butter are high in saturated fats, and low-fat versions may be lower in fats but tend to be higher in carbs. You also need to bear in mind that many dairy products are high in calories; your weight loss may stall if you eat too much cheese, for example. It's a balancing act. To help you, most high-protein diet books have guidelines to follow and it is worth sticking to their recommendations. Don't forget to count any milk you take in hot drinks.

TIP: Add berries to plain yoghurt rather than buying flavoured varieties, and blend them together gently if you don't like big chunks of fruit in your yoghurt. If you use frozen berries, you get chilled yoghurt, and if you blend the mixture for longer and add a little water, you get a chilled fruit smoothie.

Food type	Carb (g)	Fibre (g)	Cal (kcal)	Pro (g)	Fat (g)
Milk and Cream					
Buttermilk, 250ml	20.3	n/a	138	14.3	Tr
Cream:					
extra thick, 2 tbsp	1.1	–	70	0.8	6.9
fresh, clotted, 2 tbsp	0.7	n/a	176	0.5	19.1
fresh, double, 2 tbsp	0.5	–	149	0.5	16.1
fresh, single, 2 tbsp	0.7	–	58	1	5.7
fresh, soured, 2 tbsp	0.9	n/a	62	0.9	6.0
fresh, whipping, 2 tbsp	0.8	–	114	0.6	12
sterilised, canned, 2 tbsp	1.2	n/a	76	0.8	7.6
UHT, aerosol spray, 2 tbsp	2.5	–	86	0.6	8.3
UHT, double, vegetarian, 2 tbsp	1.2	0.2	92	0.8	9.3
UHT, single, vegetarian, 2 tbsp	1.4	0.1	44	0.9	3.9
Crème fraiche:					
full fat, 2 tbsp	0.7	–	113	0.7	12
half fat, 2 tbsp	1.3	–	49	0.8	4.5
Milk, fresh:					
cows', whole, 250ml	11.3	n/a	165	8.3	9.8
cows', semi-skimmed, 250ml	11.8	–	115	8.5	4.3
cows', skimmed, 250ml	11	–	80	8.5	0.5
cows', Channel Island, 250ml	12	n/a	195	9	12.8

TIP: Make a dip from feta cheese and low-fat yoghurt. Mash the feta with a fork, add the yoghurt and mix well. Then add chopped fresh mint and parsley, and stir thoroughly before serving.

Food type	Carb (g)	Fibre (g)	Cal (kcal)	Pro (g)	Fat (g)
Milk, *contd:*					
goats', pasteurised, 250ml	11	–	155	7.8	9.3
sheep's, 250ml	12.8	–	233	13.5	14.5
Milk, evaporated:					
original, 100ml	11.5	–	160	8.2	9
light, 100ml	10.5	–	110	7.5	4
Milk, dried, skimmed, 250ml	75.5	n/a	515	51.5	0.8
Milk, condensed:					
whole milk, sweetened, 100ml	55.5	n/a	333	8.5	10.1
skimmed milk, sweetened, 100ml	60	n/a	267	10	0.2
Soya milk:					
unsweetened, 250ml	1.3	1.3	65	6	4
sweetened, 250ml	6.3	Tr	108	7.8	6
Rice drink:					
calcium enriched, 250ml	24	–	125	0.3	3
vanilla, organic, 250ml	23.8	–	123	0.3	3
Yoghurt and Fromage Frais					
Diet yoghurts, 125g:					
banana	10.9	n/a	66	5.5	0.1
cherry	9.9	n/a	63	5.5	0.1
vanilla	10.4	n/a	66	5.8	0.1

TIP: Dairy products are an important source of calcium, so don't avoid them completely. Vegans may need to take supplements.

Food type	Carb (g)	Fibre (g)	Cal (kcal)	Pro (g)	Fat (g)
Fromage frais, 1 pot (50g):					
fruit	7	Tr	62	2.7	2.8
plain	2.2	–	57	3.1	4
virtually fat free, fruit	2.8	0.4	25	3.4	0.1
virtually fat free, plain	2.3	–	25	3.9	0.1
Fruit corner, 125g:					
blueberry	19.4	n/a	140	4.6	4.9
strawberry	21.4	n/a	148	4.6	4.9
Greek-style, cows, fruit, 1 pot (125g)	14	Tr	171	6	10.5
Greek-style, cows, plain, 1 pot (125g)	6	–	166	7.1	12.8
Greek-style, sheep, 1 pot (125g)	6.3	–	115	6	7.5
Low fat, fruit, 1 pot (125g)	17.1	0.4	98	5.3	1.4
Low fat, plain, 1 pot (125g)	9.3	–	70	6	1.3
Natural bio yoghurt, 125g	7	–	68	5.5	1.9
Orange fat-free bio yoghurt each	11.3	0.1	61	5.4	0.2
Raspberry drinking yoghurt, per bottle	12.5	0.1	78	2.9	1.8
Soya, fruit, 1 pot (125g)	16.1	0.9	91	2.6	2.25
Virtually fat free, fruit, 1 pot (125g)	8.78	Tr	59	6	0.3

TIP: Try using a little of a strong cheese rather than a larger quantity of a milder cheese to keep your calorie intake lower.

Food type	Carb (g)	Fibre (g)	Cal (kcal)	Pro (g)	Fat (g)
Virtually fat free, plain, 1 pot (125g)	10.3	–	68	6.8	0.3
Yoghurt drink, 125ml:					
natural	8.6	n/a	84	6.9	2.4
peach	16.2	n/a	94	3.2	1.8
Whole milk, fruit, 1 pot (125g)	22.1	–	136	5	3.8
Whole milk, plain, 1 pot (125g)	9.8	–	99	7.1	3.8
Butter and Margarine					
Butter:					
lightly salted, 15g	–	n/a	111	–	12.2
spreadable, 15g	Tr	–	112	0.1	12.4
lighter spreadable, 15g	0.1	–	82	0.1	9
Margarine, hard					
animal & vegetable fat, over 80% fat, 15g	0.2	n/a	108	–	11.9
Margarine, soft					
polyunsaturated, over 80% fat, 15g	–	n/a	112	Tr	12.4
Spreads					
Olive oil spread, 15g	0.2	Tr	80	–	8.9

TIP: If your high-protein diet requires you to count carbs accurately, don't forget to include the carbs in milky drinks.

Food type	Carb (g)	Fibre (g)	Cal (kcal)	Pro (g)	Fat (g)
Olive oil spread, *contd:*					
very low fat (20-25%)	0.4	–	39	0.9	3.8
Polyunsaturated spread:					
buttery, 15g	–	–	80	Tr	8.9
light, 15g	0.9	–	55	–	5.7
low salt, 15g	Tr	–	80	Tr	8.9
sunflower spread, 15g	–	–	95	–	10.5
Pro-biotic, 15g	0.6	Tr	50	–	5.3
light	0.2	Tr	34	0.5	3.5
Cheeses					
Bel Paese, individual, 25g	–	–	77	5.8	6
Bavarian smoked, 25g	0.1	–	69	4.3	5.8
Brie, 25g	0.1	–	76	5.5	6
Caerphilly, 25g	–	–	93	5.8	7.8
Cambozola, 25g	0.1	–	108	3.3	10.5
Camembert, 25g	Tr	–	73	5.4	5.7
Cheddar:					
English, 25g	–	–	104	6.4	8.7
vegetarian, 25g	Tr	–	98	6.4	8
Cheddar-type, half fat, 25g	Tr	–	68	8.2	4

TIP: Yoghurt is high in protein, calcium and riboflavin, and low-fat natural yoghurt gives you plenty of calcium for your calories. Some types of probiotic yoghurt claim to help lower cholesterol levels.

[4

110

Dairy

Food type	Carb (g)	Fibre (g)	Cal (kcal)	Pro (g)	Fat (g)
Cheshire, 25g	–	–	93	5.8	7.8
Cottage cheese:					
plain, 100g	3.1	–	101	12.6	4.3
reduced fat, 100g	3.3	–	79	13.3	1.5
with additions, 100g	2.6	–	95	12.8	3.8
Cream cheese, full fat, 25g	Tr	n/a	110	0.8	11.9
ail & fines herbs, 25g	0.5	–	104	1.8	10.5
au naturel, 25g	0.5	–	106	1.8	10.8
au poivre, 25g	0.5	–	104	1.8	10.5
Danish Blue, 25g	Tr	–	86	5.1	7.2
Dolcelatte, 25g	0.2	–	99	4.3	9
Double Gloucester, 25g	–	–	101	6	8.5
Edam, 25g	Tr	–	85	6.7	6.5
Emmenthal, 25g	0.1	–	93	7.3	7
Feta, 25g	0.4	–	63	3.9	5.1
Goats' milk soft cheese, 25g	0.3	–	80	5.3	6.5
Gorgonzola, 25g	–	–	78	4.8	6.5
Gouda, 25g	Tr	–	94	6.3	7.7
Grana Padano, 25g	–	–	98	8.8	7
Gruyère, 25g	–	–	99	6.8	8
Jarlsberg, 25g	–	–	91	7	7
Lancashire, 25g	–	–	93	5.8	7.8

TIP: Don't use butter for frying; choose an oil that's high in mono-unsaturated or polyunsaturated fat, like olive or rapeseed oil.

Food type	Carb (g)	Fibre (g)	Cal (kcal)	Pro (g)	Fat (g)
Mascarpone, 25g	1.2	–	104	1.2	10.5
Mature cheese, reduced fat, 25g	–	–	77	6.8	5.5
Medium-fat soft cheese, 25g	0.9	–	50	2.5	4.1
Mild cheese, reduced fat, 25g	–	–	77	6.8	5.5
Mozzarella, 25g	–	–	64	4.7	5.1
Parmesan, fresh, 25g	0.2	–	104	9.1	7.4
Quark, 25g	1	–	15	2.8	0.1
Red Leicester, 25g	–	–	101	6	8.5
Ricotta, 25g	0.5	–	34	2.3	2.5
Roquefort, 25g	Tr	–	89	5.8	7.3
Sage Derby, 25g	0.7	–	104	6.1	8.5
Shropshire blue, 25g	0.1	–	92	5.5	7.8
Soft cheese:					
full fat, 25g	0.8	0.1	63	1.5	6
light medium fat, 25g	0.9	0.1	47	2	3.9
light with chives, 25g	0.9	0.1	46	1.9	3.9
light with tomato & basil, 25g	1.1	0.1	45	1.9	3.5
Stilton:					
blue, 25g	–	–	103	5.9	8.8
white, 25g	–	–	90	5	7.8
white, with apricots, 25g	2	0.4	8	4	6.3
Wensleydale, 25g	–	–	95	5.8	8

TIP: Try having some low-carb cheese with sticks of raw vegetables at the end of your meal instead of a dessert.

Food type	Carb (g)	Fibre (g)	Cal (kcal)	Pro (g)	Fat (g)
Wensleydale, *contd:*					
with cranberries, 25g	2.3	–	91	5.3	6.8
Cheese Spreads and					
Processed Cheese					
Cheese spread:					
original, 25g	0.9	0.1	62	3.5	5
cheese & chive, 25g	1	0.1	59	3.1	4.8
cheese & shrimp, 25g	0.7	0.1	59	3.6	4.6
cheese & ham, 25g	0.9	0.1	60	3.3	4.8
cheese & garlic, 25g	1	–	62	3.9	5
light, 25g	1.7	–	43	4	5
Cheese slices:					
singles, 25g	1.9	0.1	65	3.4	3.6
singles light, 25g	1.5	–	51	5	2.8
Cheese triangles, 25g	1.5	–	60	2.6	4.9
Processed cheese, plain, 25g	1.3	–	74	4.5	5.8
Strip cheese, 25g	0.3	–	88	5.4	6.9

TIP: Try sprinkling nuts over yoghurt; toasting them intensifies their flavour. Warm a dry frying pan; while it is heating chop a few nuts and put them in the pan once it has heated up. Stir them around until they start to colour, then add to the yoghurt.

Food type	Carb (g)	Fibre (g)	Cal (kcal)	Pro (g)	Fat (g)
See also: Jams, Marmalades and Spreads For ice cream: see under Desserts and Puddings					

TIP: Full-cream milk is high in saturated fats, so go for skimmed milk instead. If you find a sudden change difficult, then wean yourself off full-fat milk by using semi-skimmed as a halfway house.

DESSERTS AND PUDDINGS

It is best to avoid prepared desserts completely when you are on a diet, whatever that diet is. Even those puddings that are labelled 'low fat' may turn out to be high in carbs when you check the ingredients, and those called 'low calorie' often include sweeteners like aspartame. Most of the high-protein diet books include recipes for homemade desserts, but the best advice is to approach all puddings with caution. If you are eating out, go for fresh fruit, or cheese served with vegetables – you often get celery – rather than biscuits. Fruit salads are another option, but restaurants may serve them in a sugary syrup.

TIP: If you find yourself craving pudding after a meal, it is likely to be a habit – and one that you can break. Try substituting fresh fruit, or a low-fat yoghurt (but check the ingredients of flavoured varieties as many contain lots of sugar).

Food type	Carb (g)	Fibre (g)	Cal (kcal)	Pro (g)	Fat (g)
Puddings					
Bread pudding, 100g	48	n/a	289	5.9	9.5
Christmas pudding, 100g	56.3	n/a	329	3	11.8
Creamed rice, 100g	16	Tr	93	3.2	2.9
Meringue, 100g	96	n/a	381	5.3	Tr
Pavlova, with raspberries, 100g	45	Tr	297	2.5	11.9
Profiteroles, 100g	18.5	0.4	358	6.2	29.2
Rice pudding, 100g:	19.6	0.1	130	4.1	4.3
with sultanas & nutmeg	16.6	0.1	105	3.2	2.9
Sago pudding, 100g:					
made with semi-skimmed milk	20.1	0.1	93	4	0.2
made with whole milk	19.6	0.1	130	4.1	4.3
Semolina pudding, 100g:					
made with semi-skimmed milk	20.1	0.1	93	4	0.2
made with whole milk	19.6	0.1	130	4.1	4.3
Sponge pudding, 100g:					
with chocolate sauce, 100g	44.6	1.2	303	5.2	11.5
lemon, 100g	50.1	0.6	306	2.7	10.6
treacle, 100g	50	0.6	286	2.6	8.4
Spotted Dick, 100g	52.7	1	337	3.4	12.6
Tapioca pudding, 100g:					
made with semi-skimmed milk	20.1	0.1	93	4	0.2

TIP: Colour-theme fruit salads, including only red fruits, for example, and use a tablespoon of Cointreau as a base.

Food type	Carb (g)	Fibre (g)	Cal (kcal)	Pro (g)	Fat (g)
Tapioca pudding, 100g, *contd:*					
made with whole milk	19.6	0.1	130	4.1	4.3
Trifle, 100g	21	Tr	166	2.6	8.1
Trifle with fresh cream, 100g	19.5	0.5	166	2.4	9.2
Sweet Pies and Flans					
Apple & blackcurrant pies, each	35.7	1	227	2.3	8.4
Apple pie, 100g	57.8	1.2	384	3.2	15.5
Bakewell tart, 100g	56.7	0.9	397	3.8	17.2
cherry bakewell, each	28.4	0.7	199	1.8	8.7
Cheesecake, 100g:	35.2	1	294	4	16.2
raspberry	31.9	0.6	299	4.7	17.2
Custard tart, 100g	32.4	–	277	6.3	14.5
Dutch apple tart, 100g	34.4	0.6	237	3.2	9.9
Fruit pie, individual:	56.7	–	356	4.3	14
pastry top & bottom, 100g	33.9	n/a	262	3.1	13.6
wholemeal, one crust, 100g	26.5	n/a	185	2.7	8.3
Jam tart, each	22.4	0.5	139	1.3	4.9
Lemon meringue pie, 100g	43.5	–	251	2.9	8.5
Mince pies, 100g	59.9	1.5	395	3.7	15.6
luxury, 100g	55.7	1.5	387	3.7	14
Treacle tart, 100g	62.8	n/a	379	3.9	14.2

TIP: Watch out for 'carb-counted' ready meals. It is still better to make your own as they often contain artificial sweeteners.

Food type	Carb (g)	Fibre (g)	Cal (kcal)	Pro (g)	Fat (g)
Chilled and Frozen Desserts					
Crème brulée, 100g	23.5	0.2	251	1.3	17
Crème caramel, 100g	20.6	n/a	104	3	1.6
Chocolate nut sundae, 100g	26.2	0.2	243	2.6	14.9
Ice cream, 100g:					
Cornish	11.3	n/a	92	19	4.4
chocolate	11.4	n/a	91	2	4.2
Neapolitan	11.8	Tr	83	1.7	3.3
peach melba	13.2	n/a	94	1.7	3.8
raspberry ripple	13.1	Tr	87	1.6	3.1
strawberry	10.5	n/a	84	1.7	3.8
tiramisu	15.2	n/a	112	2.1	4.6
vanilla	11.0	n/a	87	1.7	4.5
Ice cream bar, chocolate-covered, 100g	21.8	Tr	311	5	23.3
Ice cream dessert, frozen, 100g	21	Tr	251	3.5	17.6
Instant dessert powder, 100g:					
made up with whole milk	14.8	0.2	111	3.1	6.3
Jelly, 100g, made with water	68.9	n/a	296	5.1	–
Mousse, 100g:					
chocolate	19.9	–	149	4	6.5
fruit	18	–	143	4.5	6.4

TIP: Don't trust portion sizes when reading labels and rely on the 'per 100g' figures instead. Some portion sizes are ridiculously small.

Food type	Carb (g)	Fibre (g)	Cal (kcal)	Pro (g)	Fat (g)
Sorbet, 100g:					
fruit	24.8	1	97	0.2	0.3
lemon	32	–	128	–	–
Tiramisu, 100g	31.2	0.3	337	3.5	22.2
Vanilla soya dessert, each	16.4	1.3	80	3.8	2.3
For yoghurt, *see under Dairy*					
Toppings and Sauces					
Brandy flavour sauce mix, 50ml	38.3	–	208	3.1	4.8
Brandy sauce, ready to serve,					
50ml	8.3	–	49	1.4	0.8
Chocolate custard mix, 50ml:					
chocolate flavour	39.3	0.1	208	3.0	4.4
low fat	39.3	0.1	203	2.2	4.1
Custard, 50ml:					
made with skimmed milk	8.4	Tr	40	1.9	0.1
made with whole milk	8.1	n/a	59	2	2.3
canned or carton	7	Tr	50	1.5	2
Devon custard, canned, 50ml	8	–	51	1.5	1.5
Artificial cream topping, 50ml	16.3	0.3	345	3.4	29.3
sugar-free	15.3	0.3	348	3.7	30.3

TIP: Fresh berries and cream is a great dessert on a high-protein diet. Don't confine yourself to strawberries, either – go for an assortment of different types.

Food type	Carb (g)	Fibre (g)	Cal (kcal)	Pro (g)	Fat (g)
Maple syrup, organic, 1 tsp	4.2	Tr	17	Tr	–
Rum sauce (Bird's), 50ml	7.8	–	46	1.4	0.8
White sauce, sweet, 50ml					
made with semi-skimmed milk	9.3	n/a	76	2	3.7
made with whole milk	9.2	n/a	86	2	4.8

TIP: Make a blackberry coulis by cooking ripe blackberries very briefly in a non-stick pan over a low heat. Stir continuously, and when the berries begin to bubble remove the pan from the heat. Push the semi-stewed berries through a sieve; the resulting pure fruit purée is particularly good with a baked apple.

DRINKS

Alcohol provides 'empty' calories and most diets suggest cutting it out altogether, at least in the introductory phase, and restricting it thereafter. Beer has a relatively high sugar content so stick to a glass of wine, preferably red, as there is some evidence that a glass of red wine a day might be helpful in preventing heart disease. Only drink alcohol with food. Fruit juices and squashes do contain some nutrients, but not enough to compensate for the blood-sugar spike they produce, or their lack of dietary fibre. 'Sugar free' versions use artificial sweeteners, about which there are still many concerns; 'diet' fizzy drinks and colas may be low-carb but provide no nutritional value and the normal versions just provide a high-sugar hit. Tea and coffee are carb-free, but the caffeine they contain can have an effect on blood-sugar levels and you need to watch the amount of milk you add. Finally, most diets recommend that you drink at least 8 glasses of water a day.

TIP: Keep a small bottle of mineral water on your desk, especially if you work in an air-conditioned office, which can be dehydrating. Aim to get through 2 small bottles in a working day – one in the morning, one in the afternoon – refilling them from the tap if you wish.

Food type	Carb (g)	Fibre (g)	Cal (kcal)	Pro (g)	Fat (g)
Alcoholic					
Advocaat, 25ml	7.1	–	68	1.2	1.6
Beer, bitter, 500ml:					
canned	11.5	–	160	1.5	Tr
draught	11.5	–	160	1.5	Tr
keg	11.5	–	155	1.5	Tr
Beer, mild draught, 500ml	8.0	–	125	1.0	Tr
Brandy, 25ml	Tr	–	56	Tr	–
Brown ale, bottled, 500ml	15	n/a	150	1.5	–
Cider, 500ml:					
dry	13	n/a	180	Tr	–
sweet	21.5	n/a	210	Tr	–
vintage	36.5	n/a	505	Tr	–
Cognac, 25ml	n/a	n/a	88	n/a	n/a
Gin, 25ml	Tr	–	56	Tr	–
Lager, bottled, 500ml	7.5	–	145	1.0	Tr
Pale ale, bottled, 500ml	10	n/a	140	1.5	Tr
Port, 25ml	3	n/a	39	–	–
Rum, 25ml	Tr	–	56	Tr	–
Sherry, 25ml					
dry	0.4	n/a	29	0.1	–
medium	1.5	n/a	29	–	–

TIP: 'Diet' versions of soft drinks may contain sugar substitutes which you'd be happier avoiding, so read the information on the cans first.

Food type	Carb (g)	Fibre (g)	Cal (kcal)	Pro (g)	Fat (g)
Sherry, *contd*					
sweet	1.7	n/a	34	0.1	–
Stout, 500ml:					
bottled	21	–	185	1.5	Tr
extra	10.5	–	195	1.5	Tr
Strong ale, 500ml	30.5	–	360	3.5	Tr
Vermouth, 50ml:					
dry	1.5	n/a	55	0.1	–
sweet	8.0	n/a	76	Tr	–
bianco	n/a	n/a	73	n/a–	n/a
extra dry	n/a	n/a	48	n/a	n/a
rosso	n/a	n/a	70	n/a	n/a
Vodka, 25ml	Tr	–	56	Tr	–
Whisky, 25ml	Tr	–	56	Tr	–
Wine, per small glass (125ml):					
red	0.3	n/a	85	0.1	–
rosé	3.1	n/a	89	0.1	–
white, dry	0.8	n/a	83	0.1	–
white, medium	3.8	n/a	93	0.1	–
white, sparkling	6.4	n/a	93	0.4	–
white, sweet	7.4	n/a	118	0.3	–

TIP: When reading drinks labels bear in mind that sugar can be described in many ways. 'Corn syrup' is the one most frequently used in canned or bottled soft drinks.

Food type	Carb (g)	Fibre (g)	Cal (kcal)	Pro (g)	Fat (g)
Liqueurs					
Cherry, 25ml	8.2	–	64	Tr	–
Coffee, 25ml	n/a	n/a	65.5	n/a	–
Coffee cream, 25ml	n/a	n/a	80	n/a	–
Orange, 25ml	n/a	n/a	85	n/a	–
Triple sec, 25ml	n/a	n/a	80	n/a	–
Juices and Cordials					
Apple juice,					
unsweetened, 250ml	24.8	n/a	95	0.3	0.3
Apple & elderflower juice,					
250ml	25.5	n/a	108	1	0.3
Apple & mango juice, 250ml	25.3	n/a	108	1	0.3
Barley water, 250ml:					
lemon, original	54.5	Tr	241	0.8	Tr
no added sugar	27.5	–	28	0.5	–
orange, original	57.8	Tr	244	0.8	Tr
Blackcurrant & apple juice,					
250ml	24.3	n/a	108	Tr	Tr
Carrot juice, 250ml	14.3	–	60	1.3	0.3
Cranberry juice, 250ml	29.3	Tr	123	Tr	Tr

TIP: Fizzy drinks sometimes contain surprisingly high amounts of sodium (salt). Check labels carefully and consider choosing fizzy water instead. Try adding a splash of fresh juice to turn mineral water into a 'spritzer'.

Food type	Carb (g)	Fibre (g)	Cal (kcal)	Pro (g)	Fat (g)
Grape juice, unsweetened, 250ml	29.3	–	115	0.8	0.3
Grapefruit juice, 250ml	22	n/a	103	1.3	Tr
Lemon squash, low calorie, 250ml	1	n/a	18	–	–
Lime juice cordial, undiluted, 25ml	7.5	n/a	28	–	–
Orange & mango fruit juice, no added sugar, 250ml	2	n/a	21	0.5	Tr
Orange & pineapple fruit juice, 250ml	27.5	n/a	120	1.3	Tr
Orange juice, unsweetened, 250ml	22	n/a	90	1.3	0.3
Orange squash, low calorie, 250ml	6	–	25	0.3	–
Pineapple juice, unsweetened, 250ml	26.3	n/a	103	0.8	0.3
Tomato juice, 250ml:	7.5	n/a	35	2	Tr
cocktail (Britvic), 250ml	9	n/a	52	2.3	0.3

TIP: Dehydration can make you think you are hungry, so make sure you drink your 8 glasses of water – about 1.5 litres – a day. That quantity doesn't include caffeinated drinks, so you can't count tea or coffee, but you could include herb tea. You'll probably need to visit the toilet more frequently at first until you get used to it.

Food type	Carb (g)	Fibre (g)	Cal (kcal)	Pro (g)	Fat (g)
Fizzy Drinks					
Apple drink, sparkling, 330ml	22.4	n/a	95	Tr	Tr
Bitter lemon, 355ml	29.5	n/a	126	Tr	Tr
Cherry Coke, 330ml	36.3	n/a	149	–	–
Cherryade, 330ml	22.4	n/a	94	Tr	Tr
Cola, 330ml	35	n/a	142	–	–
diet	–	n/a	1	–	–
Cream Soda, 330ml	17.5	n/a	71	–	–
Dandelion & Burdock, 330ml	16.2	n/a	65	Tr	Tr
Ginger Ale, American 330ml	30.4	n/a	124	–	–
Ginger Ale, Dry 330ml	12.5	n/a	52	–	–
Ginger beer, 330ml	28.1	n/a	116	Tr	–
Irn Bru, 330ml	33.3	–	135	Tr	Tr
diet, 330ml	Tr	–	2	Tr	Tr
Lemon drink, sparkling, 330ml	39.6	n/a	165	–	–
low calorie	1.3	n/a	7	–	–
Lemonade, 330ml	19.1	n/a	73	Tr	–
low calorie	Tr	n/a	5	Tr	Tr
Glucose drink, 330ml	59.1	n/a	241	Tr	–
Orange drink, 330ml	22.1	n/a	96	Tr	Tr
low calorie	2.3	n/a	18	Tr	Tr

TIP: Don't forget that there is caffeine in some fizzy drinks. It causes a blood-sugar spike which you should be trying to avoid. Most high-protein diets recommend that you avoid caffeine during their introductory phases.

Food type	Carb (g)	Fibre (g)	Cal (kcal)	Pro (g)	Fat (g)
Ribena, sparkling, 330ml	43.9	–	178	–	–
low calorie	0.3	–	7	–	–
Tonic water, 330ml	20.5	n/a	86	–	–
Water, flavoured, 330ml	Tr	–	3	Tr	–
Hot and Milky Drinks					
Beef instant drink, per mug	51.3	0.3	425	54.3	0.3
Cappuccino, per sachet:					
instant	12	–	72	2	1.7
unsweetened	9.8	–	77	2.7	3
Chicken instant drink, per mug	48.8	5.3	323	24.3	3.5
Cocoa, per mug					
made with semi-skimmed milk	17.4	0.5	142	8.7	4.7
made with whole milk	17.0	0.5	190	8.5	10.5
Coffee, black, per mug	0.8	n/a	5	0.5	Tr
Coffee creamer, per tsp	3.7	–	26	0.2	2.2
virtually fat free, per tsp	4.2	–	20	0.1	0.3
Drinking chocolate, per mug					
made with semi-skimmed milk	27.3	–	183	9	5
made with whole milk	26.8	2.5	225	8.8	10
Espresso, per 100ml	10	11.5	104	15.2	0.4
Herb teas, per mug	–	–	–	0.1	–

TIP: If you're used to drinking a lot of milk, check out the Dairy listings on pages 105–6 and consider the alternatives, such as soya milk.

Food type	Carb (g)	Fibre (g)	Cal (kcal)	Pro (g)	Fat (g)
Ice tea, per mug	16.8	n/a	70	–	–
Malted milk, per mug					
made with semi-skimmed milk	71.3	1.8	460	23.5	11.5
made with whole milk	70.8	1.8	575	23	22.8
Malted milk light,					
made with water, per mug	57.8	1.5	290	11.8	3.0
Strawberry milkshake, 250ml					
made with semi-skimmed milk	62.2	–	387	17	8.5
made with whole milk	47.2	–	420	17	19.5
Tea, black, per cup	Tr	n/a	Tr	0.3	Tr

TIP: Flavoured mineral waters might sound innocent but they often contain high levels of sugar, so check ingredients carefully.

EGGS

Eggs are a great source of many nutrients – protein, polyunsaturated fats and vitamins, including vitamin E and folic acid. Omega-3 eggs are particularly high in healthy fatty acids and many people prefer to choose organic, free-range eggs for their taste and also because of animal welfare considerations. The yolks contain cholesterol, and some diets recommend cooking with egg whites only. However, recent research has shown that eating an egg a day made no difference to the chance of a healthy person developing heart disease. Cook eggs sensibly and, providing you've not been specifically told to avoid them by your doctor, they should do no harm to you or your diet.

TIP: Scrambled eggs, made properly, are delicious, especially if you use organic eggs. In a non-stick pan, heat a little butter. While that is melting, beat 2 eggs per person in a bowl with a fork. Once the butter bubbles, add the eggs to the pan and start stirring. Stir continuously as the eggs begin to cook; turn the heat down. Remove the pan from the heat just before the eggs are done to your liking – they will continue to cook in the hot pan – and serve immediately.

Food type	Carb (g)	Fibre (g)	Cal (kcal)	Pro (g)	Fat (g)
Eggs, chicken, 1 medium:					
raw, whole	Tr	–	78	6.5	5.8
raw, white only	Tr	n/a	17	4.3	Tr
raw, yolk only	Tr	n/a	59	2.8	5.3
boiled	Tr	n/a	76	6.5	5.6
fried, in vegetable oil	Tr	n/a	93	7.1	7.2
poached	Tr	n/a	76	6.5	5.6
Eggs, duck, raw, whole	Tr	n/a	84	7.4	6.1
Omelette (2 eggs, 10g butter):					
plain	–	n/a	228	12.7	19.6
with 25g cheese	Tr	n/a	475	27.9	40.3
Scrambled (2 eggs with					
15 ml milk, 20g butter)	0.8	n/a	310	13.1	28.2

TIP: A poached egg on a bed of cooked spinach is a classic, useful dish. Try adding nutmeg as well as black pepper to the spinach for a different taste.

FISH AND SEAFOOD

The high levels of Omega-3 fatty acids in oily fish like mackerel, herring, salmon and tuna are a valuable contribution to your overall diet, and dietitians recommend that they form an important part of it, whether you're trying to lose weight or not. White fish are important too, particularly as a source of protein. It is probably best to make shellfish, especially prawns, a treat; they contain cholesterol, as does squid. Avoid fish coated in batter or breadcrumbs, or which has been deep-fried – usually in unhealthy trans fats. Otherwise, go ahead.

TIP: Don't thaw frozen fish in cold water. Either thaw it at room temperature and then cook it as soon as it has defrosted, or thaw it in the fridge overnight. If you do this, then put it on a large dish so the juices don't fall on anything else. Never refreeze frozen fish unless it has been cooked first, for example as part of a soup or fish pie.

Food type	Carb (g)	Fibre (g)	Cal (kcal)	Pro (g)	Fat (g)
Fish and Seafood					
Anchovies, in oil,					
drained, 100g	–	–	191	25.2	10
Cockles, boiled, 100g	Tr	n/a	53	12	0.6
Cod:					
baked fillets, 100g	Tr	n/a	96	21.4	1.2
dried, salted, boiled, 100g	–	n/a	138	32.5	0.9
in batter, fried, 100g	11.7	n/a	247	16.1	15.4
in crumbs, fried, 100g	15.2	n/a	235	12.4	14.3
in parsley sauce, boiled, 100g	2.8	n/a	84	12	2.8
poached fillets, 100g	Tr	n/a	94	20.9	1.1
steaks, grilled, 100g	Tr	n/a	95	20.8	1.3
Cod roe, hard, fried, 100g	3	n/a	202	20.9	11.9
Coley fillets, steamed, 100g	–	n/a	105	23.3	1.3
Crab					
boiled, 100g	Tr	n/a	128	19.5	5.5
canned, 100g	Tr	n/a	77	18.1	0.5
dressed, 100g	n/a	n/a	105	16.9	14.2
Eels, jellied, 100g	Tr	n/a	98	8.4	7.1
Haddock:					
in crumbs, fried, 100g	12.6	n/a	196	14.7	10

TIP: Rub a serving bowl with half a clove of garlic, put in multicoloured salad leaves, dress with a little olive oil and lemon juice and toss lightly. Arrange some cooked king prawns on top and serve with lemon slices.

Food type	Carb (g)	Fibre (g)	Cal (kcal)	Pro (g)	Fat (g)
Haddock, *contd*:					
smoked, steamed, 100g	–	n/a	101	23.3	0.9
steamed, 100g	–	n/a	89	20.9	0.6
Halibut, grilled, 100g	–	n/a	121	25.3	2.2
Herring:					
fried, 100g	1.5	–	234	23.1	15.1
grilled, 100g	–	–	199	20.4	13
Kippers, grilled, 100g	–	n/a	255	20.1	19.4
Lemon sole:					
steamed, 100g	–	n/a	91	20.6	0.9
goujons, baked, 100g	14.7	n/a	187	16	14.6
goujons, fried, 100g	14.3	n/a	374	15.5	28.7
Lobster, boiled, 100g	–	–	119	22.1	3.4
Mackerel, grilled, 100g	–	n/a	239	20.8	17.3
Mussels, boiled, 100g	Tr	–	87	17.2	2
Pilchards,					
canned in tomato sauce, 100g	0.7	Tr	126	18.8	5.4
Plaice					
in batter, fried, 100g	12	–	257	15.2	16.8
in crumbs, fried, 100g	8.6	–	228	18	13.7
goujons, baked, 100g	27.7	–	304	8.8	18.3

TIP: Try steaming fish fillets with ginger and spring onion, and serve with soy sauce and a salad made from handfuls of crunchy bean sprouts, slivers of red pepper and spring onions.

Food type	Carb (g)	Fibre (g)	Cal (kcal)	Pro (g)	Fat (g)
Plaice, *contd:*					
goujons, fried, 100g	27	–	426	8.5	32.3
steamed, 100g	–	–	93	18.9	1.9
Prawns: shelled, boiled, 100g	–	n/a	99	22.6	0.9
boiled, weighed in shells, 175g	–	–	72	15.1	1.2
king prawns, freshwater, 100g	–	n/a	70	16.8	0.3
North Atlantic, peeled, 100g	–	–	99	22.6	0.9
tiger king, cooked, 100g	–	n/a	61	13.5	0.6
Roe:					
cod, hard, fried, 100g	3	n/a	202	20.9	11.9
herring, soft, fried, 100g	4.7	–	244	21.1	15.8
Salmon:					
pink, canned in brine,					
drained, 100g	–	n/a	153	23.5	6.6
grilled steak, 100g	–	n/a	215	24.2	13.1
smoked, 100g	–	n/a	142	25.4	4.5
steamed, flesh only, 100g	–	n/a	194	21.8	11.9
Sardines:					
canned in oil, drained, 100g	–	n/a	220	23.3	14.1
canned in tomato sauce, 100g	1.4	n/a	162	17	9.9
Scampi tails, premium, 100g	26	n/a	230	8.4	10.9

TIP: Serve cold fish with some low-fat mayonnaise , but flavour it with a dash of tabasco or a dab of sun-dried tomato paste – or both – to make it more interesting.

Food type	Carb (g)	Fibre (g)	Cal (kcal)	Pro (g)	Fat (g)
Shrimps:					
canned, drained, 100g	Tr	n/a	94	20.8	1.2
frozen, without shells, 100g	Tr	n/a	73	16.5	0.8
Skate, fried in butter, 100g	4.9	0.2	199	17.9	12.1
Sole: see Lemon sole					
Swordfish, grilled, 100g	–	n/a	139	22.9	5.2
Trout:					
brown, steamed, 100g	–	–	135	23.5	4.5
rainbow, grilled, 100g	–	n/a	135	21.5	5.4
Tuna, fresh, grilled, 100g	0.4	–	170	24.3	7.9
canned in brine, 100g	–	n/a	99	23.5	0.6
canned in oil, 100g	–	n/a	189	27.1	9
Whelks, boiled,					
weighed with shells, 100g	Tr	n/a	89	19.5	1.2
Whitebait, fried, 100g	5.3	n/a	525	19.5	47.5
Whiting:					
steamed, flesh only, 100g	–	n/a	92	20.9	0.9
in crumbs, fried, 100g	7	n/a	191	18.1	10.3
Winkles, boiled,					
weighed with shells, 100g	Tr	n/a	72	15.4	1.2

TIP: Make a fresh tomato sauce for fish by cooking a few tomatoes briefly and then, once they are soft, pushing them through a sieve. If the liquid is too watery, reheat it and reduce to the consistency you prefer. It can be flavoured with herbs like fennel, black pepper, chilli…

Food type	Carb (g)	Fibre (g)	Cal (kcal)	Pro (g)	Fat (g)
Breaded, Battered or in Sauces					
Calamari in batter, 100g	13	1.5	177	7.8	10.4
Fish cakes, 100g					
fried, each	16.8	n/a	218	8.6	13.4
Fish fingers					
fried in oil, 100g	17.2	0.6	233	13.5	12.7
grilled, 100g	19.3	0.7	214	15.1	9
oven crispy, 100g	17	0.5	236	10.5	14
Fish steaks in butter sauce, 100g	3.2	0.1	84	9.1	3.9
Fish steaks in parsley sauce, 100g	3.1	0.1	82	9.1	3.7
Kipper fillets with butter, 100g	–	–	205	15	16
Prawn Cocktail (Lyons), 100g	4.5	n/a	429	5.7	42.9
Seafood sticks, 100g	14.5	1	95	8.1	0.4
Shrimps, potted, 100g	–	–	358	16.5	32.4

TIP: Fish won't smell during cooking if you bake it in a sealed packet made from foil. Place raw fillets of fish on a generous piece of foil – more than big enough to fold over the fish. Add flavourings – a bay leaf, some fresh herbs, a squeeze of lemon juice, garlic, ginger, sliced onions: whatever you fancy. Then fold the foil up around the fish and seal the sides together firmly. Put the parcel in an ovenproof dish and bake at 200°C /gas mark 6 until the fish is cooked – check by opening the parcel carefully, then reseal and return it to the oven if needed.

FRUIT

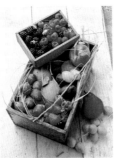

Fruit naturally contains fructose, a sugar which is quickly absorbed into the bloodstream. For this reason most high-protein diets restrict fruit consumption, or cut it out completely during the introductory phase in which you are trying to stabilise your blood-sugar levels. Don't exclude fruit from your diet for too long, however, as it contains many useful minerals and vitamins. Fruits are also a good source of fibre, so don't peel them unnecessarily – the fibre in the skin slows down sugar absorption. There can be a problem with pesticide residue on skins, so wash fruit thoroughly or buy organic. Go for unwaxed fruit, as the wax can trap pesticide residues next to the skin.

TIP: A warm lemon will yield more juice than a cold one, so leave it on a sunny windowsill for a while before squeezing it.

Food type	Carb (g)	Fibre (g)	Cal (kcal)	Pro (g)	Fat (g)
Apple, 1 medium	20.4	n/a	82	0.7	0.2
Apples, stewed					
with sugar (60g)	11.5	n/a	44	0.2	0.1
without sugar (60g)	4.9	n/a	20	0.2	0.1
Apricots: 1 fresh	3.7	n/a	16	0.5	0.1
dried, 8 halves	9.9	1.7	45	1.1	0.2
canned in juice, 100g	8.4	n/a	34	0.5	0.1
canned in syrup, 100g	16.1	n/a	63	0.4	0.1
Avocado, half medium	1.6	n/a	160	1.6	16.4
Banana, 1 medium	23.2	n/a	95	1.2	0.3
Blackberries:					
fresh, 75g	3.8	n/a	19	0.7	0.2
stewed with sugar, 75g	10.4	n/a	42	0.5	0.2
stewed without sugar, 75g	3.3	4.2	16	0.6	0.2
Blackcurrants:					
fresh, 75g	5	n/a	21	0.7	Tr
stewed with sugar, 75g	11.3	n/a	44	0.5	Tr
canned in syrup, 75g	13.8	2.7	54	0.5	Tr
Blueberries, fresh, 75g	7.6	1.6	32	0.4	0.2
Cherries, half cup fresh (90g)	10.4	0.8	43	0.8	0.09
Cherries, glacé, 25g	16.6	0.2	63	0.1	–

TIP: Fresh cherries, sorted, washed and piled in an attractive bowl, can make a simple and delicious dessert. They also provide useful amounts of vitamin C.

Food type	Carb (g)	Fibre (g)	Cal (kcal)	Pro (g)	Fat (g)
Clementines, 1 medium	6.6	0.9	28	0.7	0.1
Coconut:					
creamed, 2 tbsp	1.4	n/a	134	1.2	13.8
desiccated, 2 tbsp	1.3	n/a	121	1.1	12.4
milk, 100ml	1.6	–	166	1.6	17.0
Cranberries, fresh, 75g	3	3.2	12	–	–
Damsons:					
fresh, 75g	7.2	n/a	29	0.4	Tr
stewed with sugar (2 tbsp)	5.7	n/a	22	0.1	Tr
Dates, quarter cup (50g)	15.7	n/a	62	0.8	0.1
Figs:					
1 fresh	9.6	1.7	37	0.4	0.2
dried, ready to eat, 50g	24.5	0.8	112	1.7	0.8
canned in syrup, 100g	18	0.7	75	0.4	0.1
Fruit cocktail, 100g					
canned in juice	7.2	n/a	29	0.4	Tr
canned in syrup	14.8	n/a	57	0.4	Tr
Gooseberries:					
fresh, 75g	2.3	n/a	14	0.8	0.3
stewed with sugar (2 tbsp)	3.9	n/a	16	0.2	0.1
Grapefruit, half, fresh	7.7	n/a	34	0.9	0.1

TIP: Use lemon or lime juice to add flavour to fish dishes or casseroles, and try experimenting with lemongrass as well. It gives an exotic flavour to Thai curries and stir-fries.

Food type	Carb (g)	Fibre (g)	Cal (kcal)	Pro (g)	Fat (g)
Grapes, black/white, seedless, fresh, 75g	11.6	n/a	45	0.3	0.1
Greengages:					
fresh, 75g	6.5	1.2	26	0.4	Tr
stewed with sugar (2 tbsp)	8	0.4	32	0.4	–
Guavas, fresh, 60g	3	n/a	16	0.5	0.3
Honeydew melon: see Melon					
Jackfruit, fresh, 75g	16.1	–	66	1.0	0.2
Kiwi fruit, peeled, each	10.6	n/a	49	1.1	0.5
Lemon, whole	3.2	n/a	19	1	0.3
Lychees, fresh, 75g	10.7	n/a	44	0.7	0.1
canned in syrup, 100g	17.7	n/a	68	0.4	Tr
Mandarin oranges, 100g:					
canned in juice	7.7	n/a	32	0.7	Tr
canned in syrup	13.4	n/a	52	0.5	Tr
Mangos, 1 medium	16.3	n/a	66	0.8	0.2
Melon, fresh, medium slice:					
cantaloupe	4.9	n/a	22	0.7	0.1
galia	6.3	n/a	27	0.6	0.1
honeydew	7.5	n/a	32	0.7	0.1
watermelon	8	n/a	35	0.6	0.3

TIP: Purple and red fruits are great sources of antioxidants and berries are very low in carbs, so take your pick. Don't forget blackcurrants, which are a rich source of vitamin C.

Food type	Carb (g)	Fibre (g)	Cal (kcal)	Pro (g)	Fat (g)
Nectarines, 1 medium	13.5	n/a	60	2.1	0.1
Oranges, 1 medium	12.9	n/a	56	1.7	0.2
Papaya, half, fresh	10	n/a	41	0.6	0.1
Passionfruit, 75g					
fresh (flesh & pips only)	4.4	n/a	27	2	0.3
Paw-paw, half, fresh	10	2.5	41	0.6	0.1
Peach, 1 medium	11.5	n/a	50	1.5	0.2
canned in juice, 100g	9.7	n/a	39	0.6	Tr
canned in syrup, 100g	14	n/a	55	0.5	Tr
Pear, 1 medium	15	n/a	60	0.5	0.2
canned in juice, 100g	8.5	n/a	33	0.3	Tr
canned in syrup, 100g	13.2	n/a	50	0.2	Tr
Pineapple, fresh, 60g	6.1	n/a	25	0.2	0.1
canned in juice, 100g	12.2	n/a	47	0.3	Tr
canned in syrup, 100g	16.5	n/a	64	0.5	Tr
Plums, 1 medium	8.8	n/a	36	0.6	0.1
Prunes, canned in juice, 100g	19.7	n/a	79	0.7	0.2
canned in syrup, 100g	23	n/a	90	0.6	0.2
Prunes, dried: *see under* Snacks					
Raisins: *see under* Snacks					

TIP: An ordinary apple can be sprayed up to 16 times during its growth with as many as 36 different chemicals, and pesticides can penetrate the skin of citrus fruit, so think seriously about choosing organic fruit when you can.

Food type	Carb (g)	Fibre (g)	Cal (kcal)	Pro (g)	Fat (g)
Raspberries, fresh, 60g	2.8	n/a	15	0.8	0.2
Rhubarb, fresh, raw, 60g	0.5	n/a	4	0.5	0.1
stewed with sugar (2 tbsp)	3.4	n/a	14	0.3	–
stewed without sugar (2 tbsp)	0.2	0.4	2	0.3	–
Satsumas, 1 medium	12.8	n/a	54	1.4	0.2
Strawberries, 70g	4.2	n/a	19	0.6	0.1
Tangerines, fresh, one	8	n/a	35	0.9	0.1
Watermelon, *see under* Melon					

TIP: Many diets, like South Beach, Rose Elliot's or Atkins, limit or prohibit fruit during the introductory phase, and then reintroduce it very gradually. Do be aware that some fruits – like bananas – are high in carbs and avoid them, even when you are eating fruit again.

JAMS, MARMALADES AND SPREADS

The high sugar content of most jams and spreads is a major problem on any diet; you are trying to keep blood-sugar levels steady and these send them upwards. If you must have jam, try some of those intended for diabetics after checking which sugar substitutes they contain, or look at fruit spreads. Never buy anything where sugar is the first ingredient listed, and remember that honey will have the same effect as pure sugar. Nut butters are an option but some are high in saturated fat and all are high-calorie. Yeast extract is a great alternative, so try to accustom yourself to a savoury taste in the mornings instead of sugary marmalade.

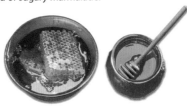

TIP: Yeast extract – Marmite – is a great source of B vitamins, and you need very little to pack a savoury punch. If you haven't tried it for a while, buy a small jar and give it a go; it could be a valuable addition to your diet. You can also use it to add extra flavour to soups and casseroles.

Food type	Carb (g)	Fibre (g)	Cal (kcal)	Pro (g)	Fat (g)
Jams and Marmalades					
Apricot conserve, 1 tsp	3.2	–	13	–	–
Apricot fruit spread, 1 tsp:					
diet	1.5	–	6	–	–
organic	1.7	0.1	7	–	Tr
Apricot jam, 1 tsp:					
reduced sugar	2.3	n/a	9	–	–
sucrose free	3.2	n/a	13	–	Tr
Blackcurrant jam, 1 tsp:					
reduced sugar	2.3	n/a	9	–	–
sucrose free	3.4	n/a	13	–	Tr
Blueberry & blackberry jam,		–	–		
organic, 1 tsp	3	0.1	13	–	–
Grapefruit fruit spread, 1 tsp	1.9	0.1	7	–	–
Grapefruit marmalade, 1 tsp	3.1	n/a	12	–	–
Honey, 1 tsp:					
clear	3.7	n/a	15	–	Tr
honeycomb	3.6	n/a	14	–	0.2
set	3.5	–	14	–	–
Lemon curd, 1 tsp	3.1	–	14	–	0.2
Marmalade:					
orange, 1 tsp	2.1	n/a	8	–	–

TIP: Consider using cream cheese, tahini (sesame seed paste), hummus or tapenade (black olive paste) as alternative types of spread.

Food type	Carb (g)	Fibre (g)	Cal (kcal)	Pro (g)	Fat (g)
Marmalade, *contd*:					
Dundee, 1 tsp	2.7	–	11	–	–
organic, 1 tsp	3.2	–	13	–	–
thick-cut, 1 tsp	3.5	–	13	–	–
Morello cherry fruit spread					
organic, 1 tsp	1.7	0.1	7	–	Tr
Pineapple & ginger fruit					
spread, 1 tsp	1.9	0.1	7	–	Tr
Raspberry conserve, 1 tsp	3.2	–	13	–	–
Raspberry fruit spread, 1 tsp:					
diet	1.5	–	6	–	–
organic	1.7	0.1	7	–	Tr
Raspberry jam, 1 tsp:	3	n/a	12	–	–
organic	3.2	–	13	–	–
reduced sugar	2.3	n/a	9	–	–
sucrose free	3.2	n/a	13	–	–
Rhubarb & ginger jam,					
reduced sugar, 1 tsp	2.5	–	10	–	Tr
Seville orange fruit spread, 1 tsp					
reduced sugar	1.5	–	6	–	–
organic	1.7	0.1	7	–	Tr

TIP: Check out the fruit spreads in your local health-food shop. Some are really inventive – pear and raspberry, for example – and they are so well-flavoured that you don't need to use much.

Food type	Carb (g)	Fibre (g)	Cal (kcal)	Pro (g)	Fat (g)
Strawberry fruit spread, 1 tsp	1.4	–	6	–	–
organic	1.7	0.1	7	–	Tr
Strawberry jam, 1 tsp:					
classic	3	n/a	12	–	–
reduced sugar	2.3	n/a	9	–	–
sucrose free	3.2	n/a	13	–	Tr
Wild blackberry jelly,					
reduced sugar, 1 tsp	2.7	0.1	11	–	–
Wild blueberry fruit spread,					
organic, 1 tsp	1.8	0.2	7	–	–
Nut Butters					
Almond butter, 1 tsp	0.3	0.4	31	1.3	2.8
Cashew butter, 1 tsp	0.9	0.2	32	1.2	2.6
Chocolate nut spread, 1 tsp	3.1	n/a	28	0.3	1.7
Hazelnut butter, 1 tsp	0.3	0.3	34	0.8	3.3
Peanut butter, 1 tsp:					
crunchy	0.8	0.3	30	1.2	2.5
smooth	0.7	n/a	30	1.3	2.4
organic	0.6	0.3	30	1.5	2.4
stripy chocolate	1.7	0.2	31	0.7	2.3
Tahini paste, 1 tsp	–	n/a	30	0.9	2.9

TIP: Experiment with alternative nut butters. You should find a selection in a good health-food shop – try almond or walnut, for example.

Food type	Carb (g)	Fibre (g)	Cal (kcal)	Pro (g)	Fat (g)
Savoury Spreads and Pastes					
Beef spread, 1 tsp	0.1	n/a	10	0.9	0.7
Cheese spread, 1 tsp:	0.4	–	10	n/a	0.7
reduced fat	0.4	–	9	0.8	0.5
very low fat	0.4	0.1	6	0.9	0.1
See also under: Dairy					
Chicken spread, 1 tsp	0.1	n/a	11	0.7	0.9
Crab spread, 1 tsp	0.1	n/a	5	0.8	0.2
Fish paste, 1 tsp	0.2	n/a	8	0.7	0.5
Guacamole, 1 tsp:					
reduced fat	0.4	n/a	7	n/a	0.6
Hummus, 1 tsp	0.6	n/a	9	0.4	0.6
Liver pâté, 1 tsp:	–	n/a	17	0.6	1.6
low-fat	0.2	Tr	10	0.9	0.6
Meat paste, 1 tsp	0.2	–	4	0.8	0.6
Mushroom pâté, 1 tsp	0.4	–	12	0.4	0.9
Salmon spread, 1 tsp	0.2	–	9	0.7	0.5
Sandwich spread, 1 tsp	1.3	–	11	0.1	0.6
cucumber, 1 tsp	1	–	9	0.1	0.6

TIP: If you're a peanut butter addict, check the brand you are using. Many contain palm oil, which helps emulsify the peanut butter and keeps it solid. Palm oil is high in saturated fat, though, and should be avoided for the sake of your health. Brands which only contain peanuts may separate but are easily stirred, and they often taste better.

Food type	Carb (g)	Fibre (g)	Cal (kcal)	Pro (g)	Fat (g)
Taramasalata, 1 tsp	0.2	n/a	25	0.2	2.6
Toast toppers, 1 tsp:					
chicken & mushroom	0.3	–	3	0.3	0.1
ham & cheese	0.4	–	5	0.4	0.2
Tzatziki, 1tsp	0.2	n/a	6	0.4	0.5
Yeast extract, half tsp	0.9	0.2	11	1.9	–

TIP: When checking ingredients, watch out for dextrose, levulose, maltose, malto-dextrin, corn syrup, glucose syrup and invert sugar – they are all forms of sugar.

MEAT AND POULTRY

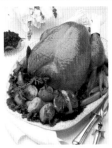

There are no carbs in either meat or poultry unless it has been processed in some way, or coated in batter or breadcrumbs. Sausages, black pudding and burgers often have carb-rich 'fillers' added, and some cold meats like ham may have added sugar or may even be cooked with honey. In addition some meat may be high in saturated fat, so trim off any visible fat and remove the skin from poultry. Deli meats, salamis particularly, can also be very high in saturates. It may be worth buying organic meat to avoid the growth hormones and antibiotics that are commonly used when raising animals for meat.

TIP: You don't have to spend a fortune on expensive cuts of meat. Cheaper ones are just as good for you, but are often better used in slow-cooked dishes like casseroles. Don't forget to trim off any visible fat before cooking, though.

Food type	Carb (g)	Fibre (g)	Cal (kcal)	Pro (g)	Fat (g)
Cooked Meats					
Bacon, 3 rashers, back (50g):					
dry fried	–	n/a	148	12.1	11
grilled	–	n/a	144	11.6	10.8
microwaved	–	n/a	154	12.1	11.7
Bacon, 3 rashers, middle (50g),					
grilled	–	n/a	154	12.4	11.6
Bacon, 3 rashers, streaky (50g):					
fried	–	n/a	168	11.9	13.3
grilled	–	n/a	169	11.9	13.5
Beef, 100g:					
roast rib	–	n/a	300	29.1	20.4
mince, stewed	–	–	209	21.8	13.5
rump steak, lean, grilled	–	–	177	31	5.9
rump steak, lean, fried	–	–	183	30.9	6.6
sausages, see under Sausages					
silverside, lean only, boiled	–	n/a	184	30.4	6.9
stewing steak, stewed	–	n/a	203	29.2	9.6
topside, lean only, roasted	–	n/a	202	36.2	6.3
topside, lean & fat, roasted	–	n/a	244	32.8	12.5
Beef grillsteaks, grilled,					
100g	0.5	n/a	305	22.1	23.9

TIP: Bacon freezes well. Buy quality bacon from a good butcher, trim it and freeze it in 2-rasher batches. Give the birds the bacon rinds!

Food type	Carb (g)	Fibre (g)	Cal (kcal)	Pro (g)	Fat (g)
Burgers, each:					
beefburgers (100g) fried	0.1	n/a	329	28.5	23.9
beefburgers (100g) grilled	0.1	n/a	326	26.5	24.4
quarter-pounder (120g)	6.1	0.5	305	17.5	23.4
chicken burger	10	0.5	140	7.5	7.9
vegetable burger	27.7	2.3	238	3.1	12.7
vegetable quarter-pounder	33.6	2.5	288	6.5	14.4
Black pudding, 2 slices, fried	29	n/a	519	18	37.6
Chicken, 100g:					
breast, grilled	–	n/a	148	32	2.2
breast in crumbs, fried	14.8	n/a	242	18	12.7
breast, stir fried	–	n/a	161	29.7	4.6
1 drumstick, roast	–	n/a	185	25.8	9.1
1 leg quarter, roast (175g)	–	n/a	413	36.6	29.6
light & dark meat, roasted	–	n/a	177	27.3	7.5
light meat, roasted	–	n/a	153	30.2	3.6
Duck, 100g:					
crispy, Chinese style	0.3	–	331	27.9	24.2
meat only, roasted	–	n/a	195	25.3	10.4
meat, fat & skin, roasted	–	n/a	423	20	38.1

TIP: Chicken breast fillets are too bland to barbecue well. Cut them into chunks, marinate them in a little lemon juice and olive oil and then thread them on to skewers, alternating the chicken with chunks of vegetables like red peppers and onions.

Food type	Carb (g)	Fibre (g)	Cal (kcal)	Pro (g)	Fat (g)
Gammon, joint, boiled, 100g	–	n/a	204	23.3	12.3
Gammon, rashers, grilled,100g	–	n/a	199	27.5	9.9
Goose, roasted, 100g	–	n/a	301	27.5	21.2
Haggis, boiled, 100g	19.2	n/a	310	10.7	21.7
Kidney, lamb, fried, 100g	–	n/a	188	23.7	10.3
Lamb, 100g:					
breast, lean only, roasted	–	n/a	273	26.7	18.5
breast, lean & fat, roasted	–	n/a	359	22.4	29.9
cutlets, lean only, grilled	–	n/a	238	28.5	13.8
cutlets, lean & fat, grilled	–	n/a	367	24.5	29.9
loin chops, lean only, grilled	–	n/a	213	29.2	10.7
loin chops, lean & fat, grilled	–	n/a	305	26.5	22.1
leg, lean only, roasted	–	n/a	203	29.7	9.4
leg, lean & fat, roasted	–	–	240	28.1	14.2
mince, stewed	–	n/a	208	24.4	12.3
stewed	–	n/a	240	26.6	14.8
shoulder, lean only, roasted	–	n/a	218	27.2	12.1
shoulder, lean & fat, roasted	–	n/a	298	24.7	22.1
Liver, calf, fried, 100g	Tr	n/a	176	22.3	9.6
Liver, chicken, fried, 100g	Tr	n/a	169	22.1	8.9

TIP: Poultry is a great source of protein, containing all the essential amino acids as well as important minerals and some B vitamins. And the fat content is low, too, especially without the skin – so always remove the skin before you cook your chicken.

Food type	Carb (g)	Fibre (g)	Cal (kcal)	Pro (g)	Fat (g)
Liver, lamb, fried, 100g	Tr	n/a	237	30.1	12.9
Oxtail, stewed, 100g	–	n/a	243	30.5	13.4
Pheasant, roasted, 100g	–	n/a	220	27.9	12
Pork, 100g:					
belly rashers, grilled	–	n/a	320	27.4	23.4
loin chops, lean, grilled	–	n/a	184	31.6	6.4
leg, lean only, roasted	–	–	182	33	5.5
leg, lean & fat, roasted	–	–	215	30.9	10.2
steaks	–	n/a	198	32.4	7.6
Pork sausages: see Sausages					
Rabbit, meat only,					
stewed, 100g	–	n/a	114	21.2	3.2
Sausages:					
beef sausages (2), grilled	14.7	0.8	313	15	22
Cumberland sausages (2)	9.8	1	215	9.9	15.2
Frankfurters (2)	2.3	Tr	369	14.1	33.8
Lincolnshire sausages (2)	18	1.3	345	14.6	23.9
pork sausages (2), fried	11.2	n/a	347	15.7	26.9
Saveloy, 100g	10.8	n/a	296	13.8	22.3
Tongue, fat & skin removed,					
stewed, 100g	–	–	289	18.2	24
Tripe, dressed, 100g	–	n/a	33	7.1	0.5

TIP: Try marinating cubes of lamb in low-fat yoghurt for 2 hours before making kebabs; it will tenderise the meat.

Food type	Carb (g)	Fibre (g)	Cal (kcal)	Pro (g)	Fat (g)
Turkey, 100g:					
breast fillet, grilled	–	n/a	155	35	1.7
dark meat, roasted	–	n/a	177	29.4	6.6
light meat, roasted	–	n/a	153	33.7	2
Veal, escalope, fried, 100g	–	–	196	33.7	6.8
Venison, haunch, meat only,					
roasted, 100g	–	n/a	165	35.6	2.5
White pudding, 100g	36.3	n/a	450	7	31.8
Cold Meats					
Beef, roasted, 50g					
silverside	1.2	Tr	69	9.6	2.9
topside	0.2	n/a	79	12.5	3
Chicken, roasted breast meat,					
50g	0.1	Tr	76	13.5	2.4
Chorizo, 50g	2	–	194	11.5	15.5
Corned beef, 50g	0.5	n/a	103	13	5.5
Garlic sausage, 50g	2.9	0.3	95	7.7	5.8
Ham & pork, chopped, 50g	0.7	0.2	138	7.2	11.8
Ham, 50g:					
canned	1	Tr	82	6	6
honey-roast	1.5	–	70	11	2.2

TIP: Veal is a low-fat meat but when eating out, remember that escalopes are frequently served coated in breadcrumbs and fried.

Food type	Carb (g)	Fibre (g)	Cal (kcal)	Pro (g)	Fat (g)
Ham, *contd*:					
mustard	0.9	–	62	11.5	1.3
on the bone	0.4	0.4	68	10.5	3
beechwood smoked	0.5	–	49	8.5	1.5
Parma	0.1	–	120	12.5	7.5
Wiltshire	0.8	0.6	101	10	6.4
Yorkshire	0.2	0.3	70	10.5	3
Haslet, 50g	9.5	0.4	72	6.5	1
Kabanos, 50g	0.5	0.3	120	12	7.5
Liver pâté, 50g	0.4	n/a	174	6.3	16.4
reduced fat	1.5	Tr	96	9	6
Liver sausage, 50g	3	n/a	113	6.7	8.4
Luncheon meat, canned, 50g	1.8	n/a	140	6.5	11.9
Pâté, Brussels, 50g	2	0.1	173	6	15.5
Pepperami, hot, 50g	1.3	0.6	277	9.5	26
Pork salami sausage, 50g	0.9	0.1	268	11	24.5
Polony, 50g	7.1	n/a	141	4.7	10.6
Pork, 50g:					
luncheon meat	1.7	–	134	7	11
oven-baked	0.7	0.4	92	13	4
Salami, 50g:					
Danish	0.3	–	302	7.8	30

TIP: Lean bacon is best. There's more meat so it's lower in fat and higher in protein – and it's also more tasty.

Food type	Carb (g)	Fibre (g)	Cal (kcal)	Pro (g)	Fat (g)
Salami, *contd:*					
German	0.5	–	198	9.5	17.5
Milano	1.5	–	214	11.5	18
Scotch eggs, 100g	13.1	–	241	12	16
Tongue, lunch, 50g	0.2	–	88	9.8	5.2
Turkey, breast, roasted, 50g	0.3	–	58	12.5	0.7

TIP: For a delicious starter, try figs with Italian prosciutto (or a similar ham). Preheat the grill and cover the grill pan with foil. Quarter the figs, remove excess fat from the ham and tear the slices into rough pieces; put them between the figs, rumpled up. Brush the figs lightly with olive oil and grill them until lightly browned. Put the grilled figs and prosciutto on a plate and drizzle with a little olive oil and balsamic vinegar. Season with black pepper and serve.

OILS AND FATS

Oils and fats are carb-free but all the high-protein diets recommend that you choose the ones that are best for your health (see pages 19–21). Go for those with the highest levels of monounsaturated and polyunsaturated fats – olive and rapeseed oils, for example – and avoid saturated fats like coconut oil, palm oil (often used as an ingredient in prepared food, from biscuits to peanut butter), lard, dripping, ghee and suet. You'll also need to bear in mind calorie content, and not use too much. Check butter substitutes for trans fat content, and try some of the olive-oil based spreads.

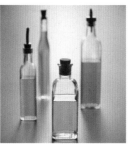

TIP: Hazelnut or walnut oils make a lovely dressing for green salads, but they shouldn't be kept for too long as they go rancid. Storing them in the fridge after opening will help extend their life a little.

Food type	Carb (g)	Fibre (g)	Cal (kcal)	Pro (g)	Fat (g)
Coconut oil, 1 tbsp	–	n/a	135	Tr	15
Cooking fat, 1 tbsp	–	–	135	–	15
Corn oil, 1 tbsp	–	–	124	–	13.8
Dripping, beef, 1 tbsp	Tr	–	134	Tr	14.9
Ghee:					
butter, 1 tbsp	Tr	n/a	135	Tr	15
palm, 1 tbsp	Tr	–	135	Tr	15
Lard, 1 tbsp	–	n/a	134	Tr	14.9
Olive oil, 1 tbsp	–	n/a	135	Tr	15
Palm oil, 1 tbsp	–	n/a	135	Tr	15
Peanut oil, 1 tbsp	–	n/a	135	Tr	15
Rapeseed oil, 1 tbsp	–	n/a	135	Tr	15
Safflower oil, 1 tbsp	–	n/a	135	Tr	15
Sesame oil, 1 tbsp	–	n/a	138	–	15.3
Soya oil, 1 tbsp	–	n/a	135	Tr	15
Stir-fry oil, 1 tbsp	0.1	Tr	122	–	13.5
Suet, shredded, 1 tbsp	1.8	n/a	124	Tr	13
Sunflower oil, 1 tbsp	–	–	124	–	13.8
Vegetable oil, 1 tbsp	–	–	135	Tr	15
Wheatgerm oil, 1 tbsp	–	–	135	Tr	15
For butter and margarine:					
see under Dairy					

TIP: Trans fats can also be called 'hydrogenated' or 'partly hydrogenated' fats, so watch out for this term on labels.

PASTA AND PIZZA

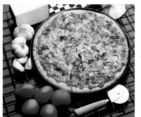 In the early stages of most high-protein diets, pasta and pizza are both out. They can sometimes be incorporated later on, but you do need to bear certain things in mind. You can minimise the impact on your blood sugar by going for wholewheat pasta served with a vegetable sauce, or a thin-crust pizza with veggie toppings. Accompanying them with green salads will help too, as will choosing pizza toppings that include olives, capers or mozzarella cheese – all of these will help to slow down the absorption of sugars from the carbs. Finally, many ready-made pasta sauces are high in sugar; check carefully before you buy.

TIP: Some dried herbs are great. Nigel Slater reckons that dried oregano is better than fresh, and the 'herbes de Provence' mixture is worth seeking out. Don't keep dried herbs for ever, though, as they go dry and musty – and they are best stored in a cupboard, out of the light.

Food type	Carb (g)	Fibre (g)	Cal (kcal)	Pro (g)	Fat (g)
Pasta					
Dried lasagne sheets,					
cooked weight 100g:					
standard	18.1	n/a	89	3.1	0.4
verdi	18.3	n/a	93	3.2	0.4
Dried pasta shapes,					
cooked weight 100g:					
standard	18.1	n/a	89	3.1	0.4
verdi	18.3	n/a	93	3.2	0.4
Fresh egg pasta, 100g:					
conchiglie, penne, fusilli	31	1.4	170	7	2
lasagne sheets	29	4.6	150	6	1.1
spaghetti	24	1	129	5	1.4
tagliatelle	24	1	129	5	1
Macaroni, boiled, 100g	18.5	n/a	86	3	0.5
Spaghetti, cooked weight 100g:					
dried, egg	22.2	n/a	104	3.6	0.7
wholemeal	23.2	n/a	113	4.7	0.9
Stuffed fresh pasta, 100g:					
four cheese tortellini	20.1	0.9	133	5.6	3.3
spinach & ricotta tortellini verdi	24	2.7	163	6	4.5

TIP: You can regulate what goes into homemade pasta sauces. For a simple one, boil, drain and purée a red and a yellow pepper, then mix the purée with low-fat fromage frais and use immediately.

Food type	Carb (g)	Fibre (g)	Cal (kcal)	Pro (g)	Fat (g)
Stuffed fresh pasta, *contd:*					
ham & cheese tortellini	13	1.7	170	6	6
cheese & porcini ravioli	21.6	2.8	164	7.8	5.2
Pasta Sauces					
Amatriciana, fresh, low fat, 100ml	5	1	155	4.4	13
Arrabbiata, fresh, low fat, 100ml	7	0.7	48	1.2	1.7
Bolognese, 100ml	2.5	n/a	161	11.8	11.6
Carbonara:					
fresh, 100ml	4.8	0.5	196	6	17
fresh, low fat, 100ml	5	0.5	81	5	4.5
Pesto:					
fresh, homemade, 100ml	6	1.4	45	2.2	1.3
green pesto, jar, 100ml	5	0.8	374	5	39
red pesto, jar, 100ml	3.1	0.4	358	4.1	36.6
Tomato & basil, fresh, 100ml	8.8	1.3	51	1.8	0.9
Canned Pasta					
Ravioli in tomato sauce, 200g can	26.4	0.6	146	6.2	1.6
Spaghetti bolognese, 200g can	26.4	1	158	6.8	3

TIP: Try spreading sun-dried tomato paste on your pizza base.

Food type	Carb (g)	Fibre (g)	Cal (kcal)	Pro (g)	Fat (g)
Spaghetti hoops, 200g	22.2	1	106	3.4	0.4
Spaghetti in tomato sauce, 200g can	26	1	122	3.4	0.4
diet, 200g	20.2	1.2	100	3.6	0.4
Spaghetti with sausages in tomato sauce, 200g	21.6	1	176	7	6.8
Spicy pepperoni pasta, 200g can	18.2	1	166	5.8	7.8
Spicy salsa twists, 200g	21.8	1.6	150	5.4	4.6
Pasta Ready Meals					
Bolognese shells Italiana, *diet*, per 100g	9.6	0.8	71	5.2	1.3
Canneloni bolognese, per 100g	11.8	n/a	149	6.1	8.3
Deep pasta bake, chicken & tomato, per 100g	13	1.3	95	4.5	3
Lasagne, each	14.6	n/a	191	9.8	10.8
vegetable, per 100g	12.6	0.9	110	5.3	4.7
Pasta bolognese, per 100g	54	n/a	375	18	9.6
Ravioli bianche, 100g	29.7	n/a	200	9.6	4.7

TIP: If you're in a pizza restaurant, limit yourself to a couple of slices and avoid deep-pan pizzas. Fill up on salads, but ask for the dressing separately, or choose your own at the salad bar.

Food type	Carb (g)	Fibre (g)	Cal (kcal)	Pro (g)	Fat (g)
Risotto, beef, per pack	57.8	5.6	346	15.3	5.9
Spaghetti bolognese, per pack	60	3.7	445	26	11
Pizza					
Cheese & onion deep filled pizza,					
100g slice	30.3	1.3	223	8.4	8.2
Cheese & tomato pizza,					
100g slice:	24.8	1.5	235	9	11.8
deep pan base	35.1	n/a	249	12.4	7.5
French bread base	31.4	–	230	10.6	7.8
thin base	33.9	n/a	277	14.4	10.3
French bread pizza, 100g slice	31	1.5	240	11	7.5
Ham & mushroom pizza,					
100g slice	29.5	1.1	227	11.4	7.5
Pepperoni & sausage pizza,					
100g slice	28.1	2.2	303	11.6	16
Pepperoni deep crust pizza,					
100g slice	29.2	1.7	263	10.6	11.5
Pizza bases, 20cm diameter:					
deep pan	56	n/a	298	8.5	4.4
standard	56	n/a	298	8.5	4.4
stone baked	55	n/a	274	8.5	2.2

TIP: As children we were told to eat up our crusts, but it is more diet-friendly to leave your pizza crust and concentrate on the topping.

Food type	Carb (g)	Fibre (g)	Cal (kcal)	Pro (g)	Fat (g)
Pizza topping, 100g:					
spicy tomato	9	1	66	1.6	2.6
tomato, cheese, onion & herbs	8.1	0.9	80	3	4
tomato, herbs & spices	9.4	0.8	67	1.5	2.6

For more pizzas: see under
Fast food

TIP: Fresh pesto can be used to accompany many dishes, not just pasta. Try it with grilled meat or fish.

PIES AND QUICHES

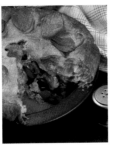

White flour has a swift effect on your blood sugar, so if you are going to treat yourself then go for wholemeal pastry and remember that all pastry-based food should only be eaten occasionally on any weight-loss programme. Don't choose anything fully encased in pastry, like a Cornish pasty, sausage roll or traditional apple pie, and choose diet-friendly quiche fillings. The potato used to top dishes like shepherd's pie or fish pie isn't the best thing for a high-protein diet, either.

TIP: You can make quiche fillings without pastry: mix the ingredients and put them in ramekins, then cook them in the oven. Standing the ramekins in a roasting tin containing enough water to come half-way up their sides will help prevent burning.

Food type	Carb (g)	Fibre (g)	Cal (kcal)	Pro (g)	Fat (g)
Chicken & mushroom pie, individual	25	1	321	8	21
Cornish pasty, each	25	n/a	267	6.7	16.3
Game pie, 100g	34.7	n/a	381	12.2	22.5
Pastry, 100g cooked:					
flaky	46	n/a	564	5.6	41
shortcrust	54.3	n/a	524	6.6	32.6
wholemeal	44.6	n/a	501	8.9	33.2
Pork pie, individual	23.7	n/a	363	10.8	25.7
Quiche Lorraine, 100g:	19.6	n/a	358	13.7	25.5
cheese & egg, white pastry	17.1	n/a	315	12.4	22.3
cheese & egg, wholemeal pastry	14.5	1.9	308	13.2	22.4
Sausage rolls, each:					
flaky pastry	25.4	n/a	383	9.9	27.6
short pastry	19.4	0.8	289	11.1	19.3
Shepherd's pie, diet 100g	10.1	0.9	73	3.5	2.1
Steak & kidney pie, canned, 100g	11.8	n/a	169	7.7	10.1
Yorkshire pudding, each	31	2.4	241	9	9

TIP: If you can't avoid pie or quiche, opt for wholewheat versions and leave the pastry from the side where it is often thicker and heavier.

RICE AND NOODLES

Rice and noodles should only be occasional treats as most varieties will have an instant effect on your blood sugar. They are both restricted on most high-protein diets but if you are going to succumb then go for brown, basmati or wild rice, and egg or thread noodles. Two level tablespoons of dry rice cooks to about 75g, the quantity given in the listings opposite. Easy-cook rice is best avoided and so are the sticky ones which generally accompany Thai, Japanese or Chinese food.

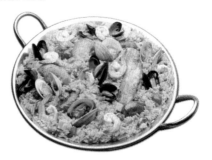

TIP: Try using bean sprouts instead of noodles in stir-fries or as an accompaniment to oriental dishes; they are very low in carbs.

Food type	Carb (g)	Fibre (g)	Cal (kcal)	Pro (g)	Fat (g)
Rice, cooked					
Arborio rice, 75g	23.3	0.3	105	2.2	0.3
Basmati rice, 75g	22.4	n/a	113	2	1.7
Brown rice, 75g	24	0.6	106	2	0.6
Egg fried rice, 75g	19.3	0.3	156	3.2	8
Long grain rice, 75g	22.6	–	103	2.1	0.3
Long grain & wild rice, 75g	27.8	–	104	3.4	0.4
Pilau rice, 75g	23	0.5	106	2.7	0.4
Pudding rice, 75g	24.2	0.2	107	1.9	0.3
Risotto rice, 75g	23.3	0.3	105	2.2	0.3
Short grain rice, 75g	26	0.7	108	2	0.3
White rice:					
plain, 75g	23.2	0.1	104	2	1
easy cook, 75g	23.2	n/a	104	2	1
Wholegrain rice, 75g	21.2	0.6	102	2.7	0.7
Noodles, cooked					
Egg noodles, 75g	9.8	0.5	47	2	0.4
Stir fry noodles, 75g	23.8	1.1	107	2.2	0.4
Thai rice noodles, 75g	26	0.7	108	2	0.3
Thread noodles, 75g	7.4	–	51	1.8	1.5

TIP: Use a non-stick frying pan or wok when stir-frying; it helps to minimise the amount of oil needed – and remember that the oil should be really hot before any ingredients are added.

SNACKS, NIBBLES AND DIPS

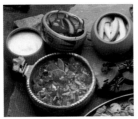

Some diets specify eating a couple of snacks a day to keep blood-sugar levels steady but between-meal hunger should be less of a problem on a high-protein diet and you may find snacks unnecessary. What you choose to snack on is critical. Most crisps and nibbles are high in carbs, salt and saturated fats, are often laden with artificial flavourings and are low in fibre; they should be avoided. Dried fruits can be another danger area; though they are much better for you, they can also be very high in carbs. Nuts are a good choice but you need to watch quantities – it's easy to eat more than you should, and salted ones should be avoided. Dips based on sour cream may be low in carbs but are high in calories, so a better choice would be a fresh salsa, hummus or tsatsiki.

TIP: For an ideal snack, tart up a tin of supermarket olives in brine. Rinse them and tip them into a bowl. Add a teaspoonful of good olive oil, some chopped fresh herbs and crushed garlic, and stir well. Alternatively, try adding a little chilli oil and some lemon zest.

Food type	Carb (g)	Fibre (g)	Cal (kcal)	Pro (g)	Fat (g)
Crisps					
Cheese corn snacks,					
per pack (21g)	11.3	0.2	110	1.7	6.3
Hoop snacks, per pack (27g)	20.5	0.6	175	1.1	9.7
Potato crisps:					
cheese & onion,					
per pack (34.5g)	17.9	1.6	176	2.1	10.7
lightly salted, 25g	13.8	1.3	121	1.6	6.7
mature cheddar with chives, 25g	13.6	1.3	120	2	6.4
pickled onion, per pack (34.5g)	17.6	1.6	173	1.9	10.6
prawn cocktail,					
per pack (34.5g)	16.9	1.5	180	2	11.6
ready salted, per pack (34.5g)	17.8	1.6	179	1.9	11.1
roast chicken, (light),					
per pack (28g)	17.9	1.7	176	2.1	10.7
salsa with mesquite, 25g	13.8	1.4	116	1.5	6.1
salt & vinegar, per pack					
(34.5g)	17.7	1.5	173	1.8	10.6
salt & vinegar, (light),					
per pack (28g)	14.6	1.4	112	1.8	5

TIP: Don't forget to watch the salt content of bought snacks; many have very high levels. In addition they are frequently high in fat, usually saturated. Try to avoid anything with more than 0.2g of sodium or 5g of fat per 100g.

Food type	Carb (g)	Fibre (g)	Cal (kcal)	Pro (g)	Fat (g)
Potato crisps, *contd*:					
sea salt with balsamic					
vinegar, 25g	13.4	1.2	122	1.7	6.9
smokey bacon, per pack (34.5g)	16.9	1.5	181	2	11.6
Quavers, per pack (20g)	12.2	0.2	103	0.6	5.8
Wheat crunchies:					
bacon flavour, per pack (35g)	19.6	1.4	172	3.4	8.9
salt & vinegar, per pack (35g)	19.1	0.9	170	3.7	8.7
spicy tomato, per pack (35g)	19.6	1.4	172	3.3	8.9
Worcester sauce, per pack (35g)	19.7	1.4	172	3.3	8.9
Nibbles					
Bombay mix, 50g	19.2	5.3	254	5.6	17.2
Breadsticks, each	3.6	0.2	21	0.6	0.4
Japanese rice crackers, 50g	39.5	0.3	200	4.7	2.6
Nachos, 100g	31	–	230	4	10
Olives, 15g black	3.4	1.7	32	0.2	1.0
Peanuts & raisins, 50g	15.9	2.4	237	8.8	15.3
yoghurt coated, 50g	27.2	1	233	4.5	12.9
Popcorn					
candied, 50g	38.8	n/a	240	1.1	10
plain, 50g	24.4	n/a	297	3.1	21.4

TIP: Try making a salsa with sun-dried tomatoes instead of fresh ones; the taste is completely different.

Food type	Carb (g)	Fibre (g)	Cal (kcal)	Pro (g)	Fat (g)
Poppadums, each:					
fried in veg oil	9.7	–	92	4.4	4.2
spicy, microwaved	10.7	3.2	64	5	0.1
Prawn crackers, 25g	10.3	0.3	77	0.2	3.9
Tortilla chips					
chilli flavour, 50g	31	n/a	248	3.5	13
cool original, per pack (40g)	25	1.4	204	3	10.5
jalapeño cheese flavour, 50g	30.5	n/a	260	3.5	13.5
pizza, per pack (40g)	23	1.4	202	3	11
salsa flavour, 50g	32.5	n/a	247	3.5	13
salted, 50g	30	2.5	230	3.8	11.3
tangy cheese, per pack (40g)	23	1.2	204	3.2	11
Trail mix, 50g	18.6	n/a	216	4.6	14.3
Twiglets, 50g	28.7	5.7	192	6.2	5.9
curry	28	3	225	4	10.7
tangy	28	2.8	227	4	2.8
Dried Fruit					
Apple rings, 25g	15	2.4	60	0.5	0.1
Apricots, 25g	9.1	n/a	40	1	0.2
Banana, 25g	13.4	2.4	55	0.8	0.2

TIP: Hummus is more than just a dip. Try it on an open sandwich – it is especially good with mustard and cress, and you won't need any butter or spread. It is also high in B vitamins.

Food type	Carb (g)	Fibre (g)	Cal (kcal)	Pro (g)	Fat (g)
Banana chips, 25g	16.2	2	133	0.4	7.4
Currants, 25g	17	n/a	67	0.6	0.1
Dates, flesh & skin, 25g	17	n/a	68	0.8	0.1
Figs, 25g	13.2	n/a	57	0.9	0.4
Fruit salad, 25g	11.1	1.8	46	0.8	0.2
Mixed fruit, 25g	17	n/a	67	0.6	0.1
Pineapple, diced, 25g	21	0.9	87	–	Tr
Prunes, 25g	9.6	1.6	40	0.7	0.1
Raisins, seedless, 25g	17.3	0.5	72	0.5	0.1
Sultanas, 25g	17.4	0.5	69	0.7	0.1
Nuts and Seeds					
Almonds:					
weighed with shells, 50g	1.3	1.4	115	3.9	10.3
flaked/ground, 25g	1.8	1.8	158	6.3	14
Brazils:					
weighed with shells, 50g	0.7	1.9	157	3.3	15.7
kernel only, 25g	0.8	1.3	170	3.5	17
Cashews:					
kernel only, 25g	4.5	0.8	144	4.5	12
pieces, 25g	4.3	0.8	156	6	12.7

TIP: Skinned, boneless sardines in olive oil or brine make an instant dip or pâté when drained and whizzed in a blender with low-fat cream cheese and a little black pepper.

Food type	Carb (g)	Fibre (g)	Cal (kcal)	Pro (g)	Fat (g)
Chestnuts, kernel only, 25g	9.2	n/a	43	0.5	0.7
Coconut: see under Fruit					
Hazelnuts:					
weighed with shell, 50g	1.2	1.3	124	2.7	12.1
kernel only, 25g	1.5	1.5	167	4.3	16
Hickory nuts: see Pecans					
Macadamia nuts, salted, 50g	2.4	n/a	374	4	38.8
Mixed nuts, 25g	2	n/a	152	5.7	13.5
Monkey nuts: see Peanuts					
Peanuts:					
plain, weighed with shells, 50g	4.3	2.2	195	8.9	15.9
plain, kernel only, 25g	3.1	–	141	6.5	11.5
dry roasted, 50g	5.2	n/a	295	12.9	24.9
roasted & salted, 50g	3.6	n/a	301	12.4	26.5
Pecans, kernel only, 25g	1.5	1.2	175	2.8	17.5
Pine nuts, kernel only, 25g	1	n/a	172	3.5	17.2
Pistachios, weighed with shells, 50g	2.3	1.7	83	2.5	7.7
Poppy seeds, 10g	1.9	–	56	2.1	4.4
Pumpkin seeds, 25g	3.8	1.3	142	6.1	11.4
Sesame seeds, 10g	0.6	0.7	64	2.3	5.8
Sunflower seeds, 25g	4.7	1.5	145	5	11.9

TIP: Nuts and seeds are excellent sources of essential fatty acids. Just don't over-indulge.

Food type	Carb (g)	Fibre (g)	Cal (kcal)	Pro (g)	Fat (g)
Walnuts:					
weighed with shell, 50g	0.7	0.8	148	3.2	14.7
halves, 25g	0.8	0.9	172	3.7	17.1
Dips					
Curry & mango dip, 100g	6.1	–	334	4.5	32.4
Mexican dips, 100g:					
guacamole	86	n/a	140	n/a	12.2
Mexican bean	12.1	2.4	89	2.7	3.3
spicy	4.8	–	324	4.7	31.7
Hummus, 100g	11.6	n/a	187	7.6	12.6
Onion & chive dip, 100g	5.6	0.5	283	4.6	26.9
Salsa, 100g					
cheese	9.3	n/a	143	2.5	10.7
cool, organic	6.3	1.2	141	1.1	0.4

TIP: For a Zone-balanced snack (see page 59), try one of the following: 15g tortilla chips with 1 tablespoon salsa, 30g low-fat cheese and 1 tablespoon of avocado; or 30g low-fat mozzarella with 85g grapes and 6 peanuts; or 60ml low-fat cottage cheese with 100g crushed pineapple and 3 almonds on top. Atkins Diet snacks can include blanched broccoli florets and carrot sticks with a sour cream dip; celery stuffed with cream cheese; hard-boiled eggs stuffed with low-carb mayo; or a small bowl of popcorn. South Beach snacks often use cos lettuce or chicory leaves to roll cream cheese or salsa inside.

Food type	Carb (g)	Fibre (g)	Cal (kcal)	Pro (g)	Fat (g)
Salsa, *contd*:					
hot, organic	6.2	1.1	141	1.1	0.4
picante	4.6	–	28	1.4	0.5
Sour-cream based dips, 100g	4	n/a	360	2.9	37
Taramasalata, 100g	4.1	n/a	504	3.2	52.9
Tzatziki, 100g	1.9	n/a	66	3.8	4.9

TIP: Blend tofu with a little tabasco and fresh herbs to make a tasty dip for raw vegetables; several scientific studies have highlighted the benefits of eating more soya, and this is a good way to do it.

SOUP

Soup can be a useful addition to any diet and clear consommés are the lowest-calorie and lowest-carb option. They can, however, be rather unsatisfying. The best soups to go for have a base of vegetable, fish or poultry stock and lots of vegetables and other flavourings, like garlic, herbs and spices. Avoid those based on cream, or thickened with potato or flour. Use pulses to thicken soups: lentils, haricot beans and chickpeas are particularly good. Always read the labels on bought soups, even the 'fresh and healthy' varieties from the chiller cabinet, and reject any that include prohibited ingredients. Don't garnish soup with croûtons, and resist having bread and butter on the side.

TIP: When you make soup, prepare extra and freeze it; that way you are creating your own, diet-friendly ready meals. The flavours of spices, herbs and salt often intensify with the length of time they are frozen, so eat spicy or salty soups fairly quickly.

Food type	Carb (g)	Fibre (g)	Cal (kcal)	Pro (g)	Fat (g)
Canned Soups					
Beef broth, 200ml	13.8	2	86	4.4	1.4
Beef consommé, 200ml	1.4	–	26	5.2	Tr
Beef & vegetable soup, 200ml	14.4	2	96	5.8	1.6
Broccoli soup, 200ml	11.8	0.8	90	2.6	3.6
Broccoli & potato soup, 200ml	11.6	1.4	62	2.6	0.6
Carrot & butter bean soup, 200ml	154	3.4	108	3.2	3.8
Carrot & coriander soup, 200ml	12	1.6	82	1.6	3
Carrot & lentil soup, low calorie, 200ml	12	1.6	62	2.8	0.2
Carrot, parsnip & nutmeg organic, 200ml	11.4	2	54	1.4	0.4
Chicken broth, 200ml	10.8	1.2	68	3	0.8
Chicken soup, low calorie, 200ml	8.2	–	60	2.4	2
Chicken & ham, 200ml	13.8	1.4	92	4.3	2
low calorie	8.8	0.9	59	1.1	2.2
Chicken & sweetcorn soup, 200ml	12.4	1.2	78	3.2	1.8
Chicken & vegetable soup, 200ml	12.2	2.4	72	3.4	1

TIP: Keep tubes of tomato, garlic and olive purée handy – they are great for stirring into soups and casseroles, or using to flavour dips.

Food type	Carb (g)	Fibre (g)	Cal (kcal)	Pro (g)	Fat (g)
Chicken & white wine soup, 200ml	7.6	n/a	94	1.8	6.4
Chicken noodle soup, low calorie, 200ml	6.2	0.4	34	1.4	0.2
Cock-a-leekie soup, 200ml	8.2	0.6	46	1.8	0.6
Consommé, 200ml	1.2	n/a	16	3	–
Cream of asparagus, 200ml	12	0.4	134	2.2	8.6
Cream of celery soup, 200ml	6	n/a	92	1.2	7.2
Cream of chicken soup, 200ml	12.2	0.2	138	3.6	8.4
Cream of chicken & mushroom, 200ml	9.2	0.2	100	3.2	5.6
Cream of mushroom, 200ml	11	0.2	126	1.8	8.2
Cream of tomato, 200ml	13.2	0.8	114	1.8	6
Creamy chicken with vegetables, fresh soup, 200ml	11	0.8	194	3.8	15
Cullen skink, 200ml	15.4	0.8	172	12.8	6.6
French onion soup, 200ml	8.6	0.8	42	1.4	0.2
Garden pea & mint fresh soup, 200ml	12.2	3	124	4.6	6.4
Italian bean & pasta soup, 200ml	15.8	2.2	84	4	0.6
Lentil soup, 200ml	14.8	2	80	4.6	0.4

TIP: Always add fresh herbs to soup towards the end of cooking – that way the flavour will come through.

Food type	Carb (g)	Fibre (g)	Cal (kcal)	Pro (g)	Fat (g)
Lobster bisque, 200ml	8.2	0.4	92	6	4
Mediterranean tomato, 200ml	13.6	1.4	66	2	0.4
Minestrone soup:					
chunky fresh, 200ml	11.8	1.8	68	2.6	1.2
Miso, 200ml	4.7	–	40	2.6	1.2
Mulligatawny beef curry soup					
200ml	14.6	1.2	94	10.4	1.8
Mushroom soup:					
low calorie, 200ml	8.8	0.2	54	2	1.2
Oxtail soup, 200ml	13	0.6	74	3.2	1
Parsnip & carrot:					
low calorie, 200ml	10.6	1.8	50	1	0.4
Pea & ham, 200ml	16.6	2.4	110	6	2.2
Potato & leek, 200ml	16.2	1.6	90	2.2	1.8
Royal game, 200ml	12.4	0.4	82	5.6	1
Scotch broth, 200ml	15	1.8	94	3.8	2
Spicy parsnip, 200ml	12.2	3	102	2.2	5
Spicy tomato & rice with					
sweetcorn, 200ml	18.4	1	90	2.6	0.6
Spring vegetable soup, 200ml	12.4	1.4	62	1.6	0.8

TIP: Chopped parsley is the classic soup garnish but experiment with some alternatives. Coriander is good on spicier soups, or try mint with pea or cucumber soups and basil with tomato. Chopped chives suit most varieties.

Food type	Carb (g)	Fibre (g)	Cal (kcal)	Pro (g)	Fat (g)
Thai chicken with noodles, 200ml	13.6	0.6	94	3.4	0.8
Tomato soup:					
low calorie, 200ml	9.4	0.6	52	1.4	1.0
Vegetable soup, 200ml	16.4	1.8	86	2	1.4
chunky fresh, 200ml	15.4	2.2	80	3.2	0.6
low calorie, 200ml	11.8	1.8	62	2	0.6
Winter vegetable soup, 200ml	16.4	2.2	92	5.6	0.4
low calorie, 200ml	12.0	1.6	62	3.2	0.2
Sachet/Cup Soups					
Beef & tomato cup soup, *per sachet*	15.8	1	83	1.4	1.6
Chicken soup, cup soup *per sachet*	8.3	1.4	83	1.1	5
Cream of asparagus cup soup, *per sachet*	18	2.3	134	0.7	6.6

TIP: Make your own vegetable stock from scratch – commercial ones often contain lots of preservatives and may be too salty. Put two garlic cloves, a halved onion, a celery stick and a carrot into a pan; cover with water. Bring to the boil and simmer for about an hour; strain carefully before use. Don't add salt or pepper while it's cooking; salt becomes too intense and peppercorns can make a stock cloudy and give it a strange burnt taste.

Food type	Carb (g)	Fibre (g)	Cal (kcal)	Pro (g)	Fat (g)
Cream of mushroom, cup soup					
per sachet	15.2	2	121	0.9	6.3
Cream of vegetable cup soup,					
per sachet	17.3	2.8	135	1.8	6.5
Creamy potato & leek					
cup soup, per sachet	15.5	3	109	1.9	4.4
Leek & potato low calorie,					
per sachet	10.2	0.5	57	0.9	1.4
Mediterranean tomato:					
low calorie, per sachet	9.6	0.7	58	1.1	1.7
Minestrone soup:					
cup soup, per sachet	16.5	1.2	98	1.6	2.8
low calorie, per sachet	9.9	1.3	56	1.3	1.2
Oxtail soup, per sachet	11.2	0.8	83	2.2	3.3
Tomato cup soup,					
per sachet	17.2	0.7	92	0.7	2.3

TIP: Most soup recipes are easily adapted to high-protein diets but if you increase or reduce the quantities in a recipe it may affect the cooking time. Check as you cook – it is best to do this anyway, as no two ovens (or cooks) are the same.

SUGAR AND SWEETENERS

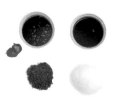

Sugar should be avoided as much as possible. One level teaspoonful contains nearly 5g of carbs and has an immediate effect on your blood sugar, producing an almost-instant spike. If you use a lot, wean yourself off it gradually by cutting down the quantity you use in drinks and avoiding sweets, cakes, biscuits and sweet puddings. Artificial sweeteners are available, but questions have been raised about the safety of some, and you may be happier avoiding them; it is probably best to train your body to do without. If you really cannot, then go for the natural sugar fructose – you'll need less as it's sweeter than sugar.

TIP: Fructose cooks more quickly than sugar. Most packs give clear guidelines on how to adapt recipes and cooking times, so make sure you check these out before using it.

Food type	Carb (g)	Fibre (g)	Cal (kcal)	Pro (g)	Fat (g)
Amber sugar crystals, 1 tsp	5	–	20	Tr	–
Date syrup, 1 tsp	3.7	Tr	15	0.1	–
Golden syrup, 1 tsp	4	–	15	–	–
Honey, 1 tsp	6.5	–	26	–	Tr
Icing sugar, 1 tsp	5	–	20	–	–
Jaggery	4.8	n/a	18	–	–
Maple syrup, 1 tsp	4.2	Tr	17	Tr	–
Molasses, 1 tsp	4	–	16	–	–
Sugar:					
caster, 1 tsp	5	–	20	–	–
dark brown, soft, 1 tsp	4.8	–	19	–	–
demerara, cane, 1 tsp	5	Tr	20	Tr	–
granulated, 1 tsp	5	–	20	–	–
light brown, soft, 1 tsp	4.7	–	19	–	–
preserving, 1 tsp	5	–	20	–	–
cube, white, each	5	–	20	–	–
Treacle, black, 1 tsp	3.3	n/a	13	0.1	–
Sweeteners					
Canderel, 1 tsp	0.47	–	1.9	0.01	–
Hermesetas, 1 tsp	0.28	0.21	1.4	0.01	–
Splenda, 1 tsp	0.5	–	2	–	–

TIP: Don't be tempted to substitute honey for sugar as it actually contains more carbs – over 6g per teaspoon.

SWEETS AND CHOCOLATES

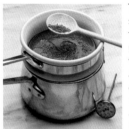

The labels on almost all sweets will reveal that they are mainly composed of sugar – just what you need to avoid. The one possible exception, and not for regular indulgence, is dark chocolate with a high cocoa content, generally 70% or over. It contains much less sugar and saturated fat, so a couple of squares – about 20g – could make an occasional treat. The rate of sugar absorption can be reduced if nuts are included but moderation is still the key. Sugar-free gums and sweets often contain artificial sweeteners and phenylaline which can have a laxative effect.

TIP: The South Beach Diet suggests stirring shelled pistachio nuts into melted 70%-cocoa-solids chocolate, spreading the mixture thinly on to a baking sheet lined with greaseproof paper and refrigerating it until firm. This works well with almonds too – but you do have to use your willpower and not eat it all.

Food type	Carb (g)	Fibre (g)	Cal (kcal)	Pro (g)	Fat (g)
After Dinner Mints:					
dark chocolate, 25g	18.2	0.3	104	0.6	3.2
white chocolate, 25g	19.2	n/a	106	0.7	2.9
Barley Sugar, 25g	24.3	–	97.3	–	–
Bonbons, 25g:					
buttermints	21.5	n/a	106	0.2	2.2
lemon	21	n/a	106	–	2.5
strawberry	19	n/a	95	–	2.3
toffee	21	n/a	105	–	2.3
Bounty, 25g:					
dark chocolate	14.4	n/a	120	0.8	0.6
milk chocolate	14.1	1.3	118	0.9	6.4
Buttermints, 25g	22.2	–	101	–	0.9
Butterscotch, 25g	22.5	–	103	–	1.4
Chocolate buttons, 25g	14	n/a	131	2	7.5
Caramels, milk & plain					
chocolate, 25g	24.1	–	123	–	–
Chewing gum:					
Airwaves, sugarfree , 5g	n/a	–	8	–	–
Doublemint, 5g	n/a	–	15	–	–
Ice White, sugarfree, 5g	–	–	9	–	–
Juicy Fruit, 5g	–	–	15	–	–

TIP: Dried fruit is useful to nibble after a meal if you have no pudding or fresh fruit – but keep the quantities small.

Food type	Carb (g)	Fibre (g)	Cal (kcal)	Pro (g)	Fat (g)
Chocolate cream, 25g	17.5	n/a	104	0.8	3.5
Chocolate éclairs, 25g	17.5	n/a	114	1	4.5
Chocolate Orange, 25g:					
dark chocolate	14.2	1.6	128	1	7.3
milk chocolate	14.5	0.5	133	1.9	7.4
Chocolate Truffles, 25g:					
with coffee liqueur	16	0.2	119	0.9	5.5
with orange liqueur	16	0.2	119	0.9	5.5
with whiskey cream	16	0.2	119	1	5.5
Chocolate, 25g:					
milk	14.2	n/a	130	1.9	7.7
plain	15.9	n/a	128	1.3	7
Chocolate, _contd:_					
white	14.6	n/a	132	2	7.7
raisin & biscuit	15.1	n/a	122	1.5	6.2
fruit & nut	13.8	n/a	123	2	6.5
wholenut	12	n/a	136	2.3	8.8
Cough sweets, 25g	23.8	–	95.8	–	–
Cream toffees, assorted, 25g	18.3	–	108	0.9	3.5
Cream eggs, 25g	17.8	n/a	111	0.8	4
Crunchie, 25g	18	n/a	118	1	4.5

TIP: The figures in the listings are for 25g of each sweet – the smallest size sold of many varieties of chocolate bar or packs of sweets. Check the weights carefully before deciding to indulge yourself.

Food type	Carb (g)	Fibre (g)	Cal (kcal)	Pro (g)	Fat (g)
Dairy toffee, 25g	18.8	–	118	0.5	4.6
Double Decker, 25g	16.3	n/a	116	1.3	5.3
Energy Tablets, 25g					
glucose	22.3	n/a	90	Tr	–
orange	22.3	n/a	90	Tr	–
lemon	22.2	n/a	90		–
Flake bar, 25g	13.8	n/a	131	2	7.8
Fruit gums, 25g	19.3	n/a	84	1.5	–
Fruit pastilles, 25g	20.9	–	88	1.1	–
Fudge, 25g	18.3	n/a	109	0.8	3.8
Galaxy (Mars), 25g:					
chocolate	14.2	–	133	2.3	7.5
caramel	15	–	122	1.3	6.3
double nut & raisin	13.9	–	134	13.9	7.7
hazelnut	12.1	–	143	1.9	9.7
praline	13	–	145	1.3	9.9
Jellies, assorted, 25g	23.5	n/a	95	–	–
Kit Kat, 25g:					
4-finger	15.4	0.3	127	1.5	6.6
Chunky	15.2	0.3	130	1.4	7
Lion Bar, 25g	16.9	0.2	122	1.2	5.6

TIP: Pumpkin seeds are an excellent source of zinc, which is essential for a strong immune system. Try them instead of sweets when you feel the need for a little something.

Food type	Carb (g)	Fibre (g)	Cal (kcal)	Pro (g)	Fat (g)
Liquorice Allsorts, 25g	19	n/a	88	0.5	1.3
M & Ms, 25g:					
chocolate	17.4	0.7	123	1.3	5.4
peanut	14.6	0.5	130	2.6	6.8
Maltesers, 25g	14.7	0.3	121	2.2	6
Mars Bar, 25g	17.3	0.3	112	1.1	4.4
Minstrels, 25g	17.8	n/a	127	1.3	5.6
Milky Way, 25g	18.7	0.4	110	0.9	3.5
Mint Crisp, 25g	16.4	1	121	0.9	5.8
Mint humbugs, 25g	22.4	–	103	0.2	1.5
Mint imperials, 25g	24.5	n/a	99	–	–
Munchies, 25g:					
original	158	0.1	122	1.3	6
mint	16.9	0.4	108	1	4.1
Orange Cream, 25g	18	n/a	105	0.8	3.5
Pear Drops, 25g	24	n/a	96	–	–
Peppermints, 25g	25.7	n/a	98	0.1	0.2
Peppermint Cream, 25g	18.3	n/a	106	0.8	3.5
Picnic, 25g	14.8	n/a	118	1.8	5.8
Pineapple chunks, 25g	21	0.9	87	–	Tr
Polos: *mints*, 25g	24.6	–	101	–	0.3
sugar-free , 25g	24.8	–	60	–	–

TIP: An extra advantage of dark chocolate with over 70% cocoa is that the taste is so intense you shouldn't be tempted to eat so much.

Food type	Carb (g)	Fibre (g)	Cal (kcal)	Pro (g)	Fat (g)
Pontefract cakes, 25g	16.7	0.6	70	0.6	0.1
Poppets, 25g:					
peanut	9.3	n/a	136	4.1	9.3
raisins	16.5	n/a	102	1.2	3.5
Refreshers, 25g	22.5	n/a	94	–	–
Revels, 25g	16.5	n/a	119	1.3	5.2
Ripple, 25g	14.8	n/a	132	1.7	7.3
Rolo, 25g	17.1	0.1	118	0.8	5.1
Sherbet Lemons, 25g	23.5	–	96	–	–
Snickers, 25g	8.8	0.3	70	1	3.5
Spearmints, Extra Strong, 25g	24.8	n/a	99	–	–
Sugared almonds, 25g	19.5	0.6			
Sweets, boiled, 25g	21.8	n/a	82	Tr	Tr
Toblerone, 25g	14.5	0.7	133	1.4	7.6
Toffees, mixed, 25g	16.7	n/a	107	0.6	4.7
Toffee Crisp, 25g	15.2	0.2	128	1.1	7
Topic, 25g	15.1	0.4	126	1.6	6.6
Tunes, 25g	24.5	n/a	98	–	–
Turkish Delight, 25g	18.3	n/a	91	0.5	1.8
Twix, 25g	15.9	0.4	123	1.2	6.1
Walnut whip, vanilla, 25g	15.2	0.2	124	1.5	6.4
Wine gums 25g	19.2	n/a	83	1.5	Tr

TIP: Keeping blood-sugar levels steady won't just help your diet – mood swings are another symptom of blood-sugar imbalance.

VEGETABLES

Not all vegetables are equally good for your high-protein diet. Avoid starchy ones or eat them sparingly – these include potatoes, cassava, beets, parsnips and winter squashes. If you do eat them, keep your portion sizes small. Green vegetables, onions, aubergines, mushrooms and salad leaves are all fine. Tomatoes, carrots and green peas do have a higher

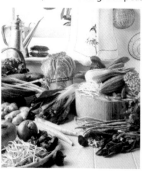

GI and so some high-protein diets limit them, but at the same time they are valuable sources of nutrients. Opt for fresh or frozen vegetables rather than canned ones.

TIP: Make a leaf salad more substantial by adding some cooked chick-peas, olives or baby broad beans. Dry-roasted pine nuts make a good garnish, particularly for a salad including olives. Using stronger-tasting leaves like rocket or watercress alongside more neutral ones like lamb's lettuce helps give green salads an extra zip.

Food type	Carb (g)	Fibre (g)	Cal (kcal)	Pro (g)	Fat (g)
Artichokes, 1 globe	2.7	–	18	2.8	0.2
Artichoke, Jerusalem, boiled, 90g	9.5	–	37	1.4	0.1
Asparagus, 6 spears, boiled	1.1	n/a	21	2.7	0.6
Aubergine, half medium, fried	1.4	n/a	151	0.6	16
Avocado, half	1.6	n/a	160	1.6	16.4
Bamboo shoots, raw, 75g	0.8	0.2	5	0.5	0.1
Beans, broad, boiled, 75g	8.8	n/a	61	5.9	0.5
Beans, French, 100g boiled	4.7	n/a	25	1.7	0.1
Beans, runner, 50g, trimmed, boiled	1.2	n/a	9	0.6	0.3
Beansprouts, mung, 25g:					
raw	1	n/a	8	0.7	0.1
stir-fried in blended oil	0.6	n/a	18	0.5	1.5
Beetroot, 90g:					
pickled	23.4	n/a	98	0.9	0.1
boiled	8.6	n/a	41	2.1	0.1
Broccoli, florets, boiled, 60g	0.7	n/a	14	1.9	0.5
Brussels sprouts, 6 trimmed, boiled	4.9	n/a	49	4.1	1.8

TIP: For a simple salad, mix peeled and cubed cucumber with seasoned low-fat yoghurt and chopped fresh mint; this gives a Middle Eastern touch when served with grilled meat, especially lamb.

Food type	Carb (g)	Fibre (g)	Cal (kcal)	Pro (g)	Fat (g)
Cabbage (Savoy, Summer), 75g:					
trimmed	3.1	n/a	20	1.3	0.3
shredded & boiled	1.7	n/a	12	0.8	0.3
Spring greens, raw	2.3	n/a	25	2.3	0.8
Spring greens, boiled	1.2	n/a	15	1.4	0.5
white	3.7	1.6	20	1.0	0.2
Carrot:					
1 medium, raw	7.9	n/a	35	0.6	0.3
1 medium, raw (young)	6.8	n/a	34	0.8	0.6
grated, 40g	3.2	1	15	0.2	0.1
boiled (frozen), 80g	3.8	1.8	18	0.3	0.2
boiled (young), 80g	3.5	n/a	18	0.5	0.3
Cassava, 100g:					
baked	40.1	1.7	155	0.7	0.2
boiled	33.5	1.4	130	0.5	0.2
Cauliflower, 100g:					
raw	3.0	n/a	34	3.6	0.9
boiled	2.1	n/a	28	2.9	0.9
Celeriac, 100g:					
flesh only, raw	5	0.4	29	1.3	0.4
flesh only, boiled	1.9	3.2	15	0.9	0.5

TIP: Try steaming vegetables rather than boiling them. They lose almost half their nutrients when boiled, but only 15% – or even less – when steamed. If you do boil your veg, be careful not to overcook them.

Food type	Carb (g)	Fibre (g)	Cal (kcal)	Pro (g)	Fat (g)
Celery, 100g:					
stem only, raw	0.9	n/a	7	0.5	0.2
stem only, boiled	0.8	n/a	8	0.5	0.3
Chicory, 100g	2.8	n/a	11	0.5	0.6
Corn-on-the-cob:					
boiled, 1 medium cob	13.3	n/a	76	2.9	1.6
mini corncobs, boiled, 100g	2.7	2.0	24	2.5	0.4
See also: Sweetcorn					
Courgettes (zucchini):					
trimmed, 50g	0.9	n/a	9	0.9	0.2
trimmed, boiled, 75g	1.5	n/a	14	1.5	0.3
trimmed, baked, 75g	1	n/a	16	1.1	0.2
fried in corn oil, 75g	2	n/a	47	2	3.6
Cucumber, trimmed, 75g	1.1	n/a	8	0.5	0.1
Eggplant: *see* Aubergine					
Fennel, Florence:					
boiled, 75g	1.1	n/a	8	0.7	0.2
Garlic, half tsp purée or					
1 clove, crushed	1.8	0.9	60	0.4	5.7
Gherkins					
pickled, 75g	2	n/a	11	0.7	0.1
Ginger root, half tsp, grated	1	0.1	–	–	–

TIP: Take tight packaging off fresh vegetables when you get them home and store them in the fridge in food bags so they keep longer.

Food type	Carb (g)	Fibre (g)	Cal (kcal)	Pro (g)	Fat (g)
Greens, spring: *see Cabbage*					
Gumbo: *see Okra*					
Kale, curly, 40g:					
raw	0.6	n/a	13	1.4	0.6
shredded, boiled	0.4	n/a	10	1	0.4
Kohlrabi, 85g:					
raw	3.1	1.9	20	1.4	0.2
boiled	2.6	1.6	15	1.0	0.2
Ladies' Fingers: *see Okra*					
Leeks:					
trimmed, 60g	1.7	n/a	13	1.0	0.3
chopped, boiled, 100g	2.6	n/a	21	1.2	0.7
Lettuce, 1 cup (30g):					
green	0.5	n/a	4	0.2	0.2
iceberg	0.6	n/a	4	0.2	0.1
mixed leaf	0.9	0.8	5	0.3	–
Mediterranean salad leaves	0.9	0.5	6	0.3	0.1
spinach, rocket & watercress	0.4	0.4	7.5	0.9	0.3
Mange-tout, 50g:					
raw	2.1	n/a	16	1.8	0.1
boiled	1.7	n/a	13	1.6	0.1
stir-fried	1.8	n/a	36	1.9	2.4

TIP: Bake large mushrooms with a little fresh pesto or olive oil and crushed garlic in the centre, and serve with grilled meats.

Food type	Carb (g)	Fibre (g)	Cal (kcal)	Pro (g)	Fat (g)
Marrow:					
flesh only, 50g	1.1	n/a	6	0.3	0.1
flesh only, boiled, 75g	1.2	n/a	7	0.3	0.2
Mooli: see Radish, white					
Mushrooms, common, 40g:					
raw	0.2	n/a	5	0.7	0.2
boiled	0.2	0.4	4	0.7	0.1
fried in oil	0.1	n/a	63	1	6.5
canned	Tr	0.5	5	0.8	0.2
Mushrooms, oyster, 30g	–	0.1	2	0.5	0.1
Mushrooms, shiitake:					
boiled, 40g	4.9	–	22	0.6	0.1
dried, 20g	12.8	–	59	1.9	0.2
Neeps (Scotland): see Swede					
Okra (gumbo, ladies' fingers):					
raw, 25g	2	–	10	0.5	–
boiled, 30g	0.8	n/a	8	0.8	0.3
stir-fried, 30g	1.3	n/a	81	1.3	7.8
Onions:					
raw, flesh only, 30g	2.4	n/a	11	0.4	0.1
boiled, 40g	1.5	0.3	7	0.2	–
cocktail, drained, 40g	1.2	n/a	6	0.2	–

TIP: Baby spinach leaves contain many more nutrients than lettuce and add a stronger flavour to salads. Older spinach is best cooked.

Food type	Carb (g)	Fibre (g)	Cal (kcal)	Pro (g)	Fat (g)
Onions, contd:					
fried in vegetable oil, 40g	5.6	n/a	66	0.9	4.5
pickled, drained, 40g	2.0	n/a	10	0.4	0.1
Parsnips, trimmed, peeled, boiled, 80g	10.3	n/a	53	1.3	1.0
Peas:					
no pod, 75g	8.5	n/a	62	5.1	1.1
boiled, 90g	9.0	n/a	71	6.0	1.4
canned, 90g	12.2	n/a	72	4.8	0.8
Peas, mushy, canned, 100g	13.8	n/a	81	5.8	0.7
Peas, processed, canned, 100g	17.5	n/a	99	6.9	0.7
See also: Petit pois					
See also under: Beans, Pulses and Cereals					
Peppers:					
green, raw, 40g	1.0	n/a	6	0.3	0.1
green, boiled, 50g	1.3	n/a	9	0.5	0.2
red, raw, 40g	2.6	n/a	13	0.4	0.2
red, boiled, 50g	3.5	n/a	17	0.6	0.2
yellow, raw, 40g	2.1	0.7	10	0.5	0.1
chilli, 15g	0.1	n/a	3	0.4	0.1

TIP: If you're making a salad using avocado, then always add some lemon juice to the dressing. It will help to prevent the avocado from discolouring.

Food type	Carb (g)	Fibre (g)	Cal (kcal)	Pro (g)	Fat (g)
Peppers, *contd*:					
jalapeños, 15g	0.5	n/a	3.3	0.2	0.1
Petit pois:					
fresh, 75g	13.1	3.1	75	5.2	0.6
frozen, boiled, 100g	5.5	n/a	49	5	0.9
Potatoes, Chips and Fries					
Chips, 150g:					
crinkle cut, frozen, fried	50.1	n/a	435	5.4	25
French fries, retail	51	n/a	420	5	23.3
homemade, fried	45.2	n/a	284	5.9	10.1
microwave chips	48.2	n/a	332	5.4	14.4
oven chips	44.7	n/a	243	4.8	6.3
straight cut, frozen, fried	54	n/a	410	6.2	20.3
Croquettes, fried in oil, 100g	21.6	n/a	214	3.7	13.1
Hash browns, 100g	26.8	n/a	153	2.9	5
Mashed potato, instant, 125g:					
made with semi-skimmed milk	18.5	1.3	88	3	1.5
made with skimmed milk	18.5	1.3	83	3	0.1
made with water	16.9	n/a	71	1.9	0.1
made up with whole milk	18.5	1.2	95	3	1.5
Potato fritters, 100g	16.3	1.2	145	2	8
Potato waffles, 100g	30.3	n/a	200	3.2	8.2

TIP: Frozen vegetables are just as good as fresh in nutritional terms.

Food type	Carb (g)	Fibre (g)	Cal (kcal)	Pro (g)	Fat (g)
Potatoes, new, 100g:					
boiled, peeled	17.8	n/a	75	1.5	0.3
boiled in skins	15.4	n/a	66	1.4	0.3
canned	15.1	n/a	63	1.5	0.1
Potatoes, old, 90g:					
baked, flesh & skin	28.5	n/a	122	3.5	0.2
baked, flesh only	16.2	n/a	69	2.0	0.1
boiled, peeled	15.3	n/a	65	1.6	0.1
mashed with butter & milk	14	n/a	94	1.6	3.9
roast in oil/lard	23.3	n/a	134	2.6	4.0
Pumpkin, flesh only, boiled, 75g	1.7	n/a	10	0.5	0.2
Radicchio, 30g	0.5	0.5	4	0.4	0.1
Radish, red, 6	1.1	n/a	7	0.4	0.1
Radish, white/mooli, 20g	0.6	–	3	0.2	–
Ratatouille, canned, 115g	8.1	1.2	58	1.2	2.3
Salsify:					
flesh only, raw, 40g	4.1	1.3	11	0.5	0.1
flesh only, boiled, 50g	4.3	1.8	12	0.6	0.2
Shallots, 30g	1.0	n/a	6	0.5	0.1
Spinach:					
raw, one cup, 30g	0.5	n/a	8	0.8	0.2
boiled, 90g	0.7	n/a	17	2.0	0.7
frozen, boiled, 90g	0.5	n/a	19	2.8	0.7
Spring onions, bulbs & tops, 30g	0.9	n/a	7	0.6	0.2

Food type	Carb (g)	Fibre (g)	Cal (kcal)	Pro (g)	Fat (g)
Sprouts: see Brussels Sprouts					
Squash:					
flesh only, 50g	1.1	n/a	6	0.3	0.1
flesh only, boiled, 75g	1.2	n/a	7	0.3	0.2
Swede, flesh only, boiled, 90g	2.1	n/a	10	0.3	0.1
Sweet potato, boiled, 90g	18.5	n/a	76	1.0	0.3
Sweetcorn, kernels, 80g:					
canned, drained, re-heated	21.3	n/a	98	2.3	1.0
canned, no salt, no sugar	13.4	2	62	2.1	–
Tomatoes:					
1 medium	4.7	0.6	29	1.1	0.6
canned, whole, 100g	3	n/a	16	1	0.1
cherry, 6	5.3	1.7	31	1.2	0.5
1 medium, fried in oil	7.5	n/a	137	1.1	11.6
sun-dried, 30g	3.3	2	63	1.3	4.9
paste, 2 tbsp	5	n/a	27	1.7	0.1
passata, 200g	9	0.4	50	2.8	0.2
chopped, canned, 200g	7	n/a	44	2.2	0.8
Turnip, flesh only, boiled, 60g	1.2	n/a	7	0.4	0.1
Water chestnuts, canned, 40g	1.9	1	11	0.7	0.1
Yam, flesh only, boiled, 90g	29.7	n/a	120	1.5	0.3
Zucchini: see Courgettes					

TIP: Tweak the bitter green shoot out of a garlic clove before use.

VEGETARIAN

Many of the high-protein diets are hard for vegetarians to follow, but Rose Elliot has stepped into the gap with a diet that boosts protein intake, as many vegetarians may not eat enough. Soya protein is one area where vegetarians have a clear advantage. It is good for everyone – the US Food and Drug Administration has recently recommended that people should eat 25g of soya protein every day – and vegetarians are much more accustomed to using soya or tofu in appetising ways. It is worth being careful with some vegetarian versions of traditionally non-vegetarian food: many vegetarian cheeses are high in carbs, for example.

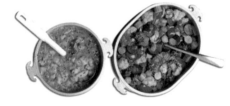

TIP: Tofu is both low in carbs and a great source of protein but flavoured tofu might contain ingredients that boost the carb count. Check the labels carefully.

Food type	Carb (g)	Fibre (g)	Cal (kcal)	Pro (g)	Fat (g)
Baked beans with vegetable sausages, 200g	24.4	5.8	210	12	7.2
Burgers:					
brown rice & tofu burgers, each	10.1	3.2	184	12.2	10.6
carrot, peanut & onion burgers, each	23.5	4.0	251	8.9	13.5
organic vegeburgers, each	27.7	2.3	238	3.1	12.7
savoury burgers, each	9.9	2.6	162	11.1	8.6
soya and black bean burgers, each	11.7	4.5	158	9.5	8.1
spicy bean burgers, each	30.9	7.6	234	7.3	9.9
vegetable burgers, each	20.8	1.7	179	2.3	9.6
Cauliflower cheese, 100g	22	–	365	18	23
Cheese, vegetarian:					
Double Gloucester , 25g	–	–	101	6.2	8.5
mild Cheddar, 25g	–	–	103	6.4	8.6
Red Leicester, 25g	–	–	100	8.1	8.4
Cornish pasty, each	37.3	2.0	452	11	28.9
Falafel, 4 (100g)	23.3	7.6	220	8	10.5

TIP: If you use soya milk, then go for one with added calcium and avoid the sweetened and flavoured ones completely. At 1.3g carbs per 250ml, it is much more high-protein-diet-friendly than skimmed milk, which has 11g carbs per 250ml.

Food type	Carb (g)	Fibre (g)	Cal (kcal)	Pro (g)	Fat (g)
Hummus, 2 tbsp	3.3	n/a	53	2.2	3.6
Lentils, 115g:					
green/brown, boiled	19.4	n/a	121	10.1	0.8
red, split, boiled	20.1	n/a	115	8.7	0.5
Macaroni cheese, individual	67	2.4	470	17	15
Nut roast, 100g:					
courgette & spiced tomato	12.5	4.9	208	11.7	12.3
leek, cheese & mushroom	13.2	4.1	240	13.2	14.9
Onions & garlic sauce, 100g	7.7	0.9	37	1.4	0.1
Pâté, 50g:					
chickpea & black olive	7.8	2.2	90	3.1	5.2
herb	3.0	–	83	3.5	8
herb & garlic	3.5	n/a	109	3.5	9
mushroom	3	n/a	107	3.5	9
red & green pepper	4.5	–	111	3	9
spinach, cheese & almond	3.2	1.2	86	3.6	6.6
Polenta, ready-made, 100g	15.7	n/a	72	1.6	0.3
Quorn, myco-protein, 100g	1.9	–	92	14.1	3.2
Ravioli in tomato sauce,					
(meatfree), 200g	26.4	0.6	146	6.2	1.6

TIP: Buy tomato purée in a tube rather than a tin – once opened, the tube will keep well in the fridge but it's difficult to make a partly used tin airtight enough. You only need a little when you're cooking as too much can give dishes a sour flavour.

Food type	Carb (g)	Fibre (g)	Cal (kcal)	Pro (g)	Fat (g)
Red kidney beans:					
small can (200g)	27	12.8	182	16.2	1
boiled, 115g	20	n/a	118	9.7	0.6
Rice drink, 240ml:					
calcium enriched	23	–	120	0.2	2.9
vanilla	22.8	–	118	0.2	2.9
Roast vegetable & tomato					
pasta, 97% fat-free, each	56	–	300	10	3.7
'Sausage' rolls, 100g	28.2	2.5	273	9.7	13.5
'Sausages', 100g (2 sausages)	8.6	1.2	252	23.2	13.8
spicy Moroccan	12.7	4.0	147	9.1	8.4
tomato & basil	9.3	3.2	147	8.6	9.8
Soya bean curd: *see* Tofu					
Soya chunks:					
flavoured, 100g	35	4	345	50	1
unflavoured, 100g	35	4	345	50	1
Soya curd: *see* Tofu					
Soya flour:					
full fat, 100g	23.5	n/a	447	36.8	23.5
low fat, 100g	28.2	n/a	352	45.3	7.2
Soya milk:					
banana flavour, 240ml	25.2	2.9	180	8.6	5

TIP: Fresh tofu will keep in the fridge for up to three days if it is stored in water. Change the water daily.

Food type	Carb (g)	Fibre (g)	Cal (kcal)	Pro (g)	Fat (g)
Soya milk, *contd*:					
chocolate flavour, 240ml	25.7	2.9	194	9.1	5.8
strawberry flavour, 240ml	18.5	2.9	154	8.6	5
sweetened, 240ml	6	Tr	103	7.4	5.8
unsweetened, 240ml	1.2	1.2	62	5.8	3.8
Soya mince:					
flavoured, 100g	35	4	345	50	1
unflavoured, 100g	35	4	345	50	1
Spaghetti 'bolognese', (meatfree) 200g	26.2	1.4	172	6.2	4.8
Sweet pepper sauce, 100g	4.3	0.5	89	1.5	7.2
Tofu (soya bean curd), 100g:					
smoked	1.0	0.3	148	16	8.9
steamed	0.7	n/a	73	81	4.2
steamed, fried	2	n/a	261	23.5	17.7
tangy, marinated	2.0	0.4	70	7.9	3.4
Vegetable biryani, each	74	–	690	12	38
Vegetable granulated stock, 30g	12	0.3	60	2.6	0.2
Vegetable gravy granules, 50g	29.7	1.6	155	4.2	2.1
Vegetable sauce, 100ml	7	2.5	59	2	2.6
Vegetable stock cubes, each	1.4	Tr	45	1.4	4.1

TIP: If you are vegetarian or vegan, remember to watch your vitamin B intake. You may need to take vitamin B12 supplements, as it is only found in animal fats.

Food type	Carb (g)	Fibre (g)	Cal (kcal)	Pro (g)	Fat (g)
Vegetable pasty, each	29.9	1.8	188	4.4	5.7
Yoghurt-tofu organic, 100ml:					
peach & mango	20.5	1.5	128	4.8	2.8
red cherry	20.1	1.5	125	4.8	2.8
strawberry	19.5	0.3	135	4.8	0.3-

TIP: You can add a burst of flavour – and useful nutrients – to vegetarian dishes by adding a little yeast extract during cooking.

FAST FOOD

If you're opting for fast food and still hoping to lose weight you must be selective. Go for salads but avoid creamy dressings; discard burger buns and remove any bread or batter coatings. Hot dogs are out, as are tomato ketchup and brown sauce – they're both packed with sugar – but mustard and dill pickles are fine. Milkshakes and fizzy drinks will have a terrible effect on your blood sugar, and your only safe drink option is likely to be still water.

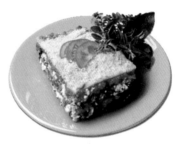

TIP: Always, always discard burger buns. Make it automatic – and never order anything extra large or super-sized, whether you're intending to avoid the bun or not.

Food type	Carb (g)	Fibre (g)	Cal (kcal)	Pro (g)	Fat (g)
Burgers/Hotdogs					
BBQ pork in a bun	67.9	3.6	555	30.2	19.4
Bacon & egg in a bun	32.3	1.7	345	18.8	15.49
Bacon in a bun	32.3	1.7	230	10.3	6.7
Bacon cheeseburger	32.3	1.7	345	19.1	15.3
Cheeseburger, each	33.1	2.5	315	16.7	13.1
Frankfurter:					
in a bun	33.5	2.2	410	21.8	22.4
in a bun with cheese	33.5	2.2	455	21.8	25.9
Half-pounder	42.3	6.7	840	51.2	51.5
Hamburger (85g)	32.8	2.5	253	13.1	7.7
Quarter-pounder	37.1	3.7	423	25.7	19
with cheese	37.5	3.7	516	31.2	26.7
Spicy beanburger	68.7	16.9	520	16.1	22
Veggie burger	46	7	420	23	16
Chicken					
Chicken chunks & chips	79.9	4.2	770	27.4	38
Chicken dunkers, portion	4.3	0.2	55	4.1	2.4
Chicken in a bun	42	1.9	435	16.3	22.2
Chicken nuggets (6)	7.9	1	208	14.2	13.3

TIP: Watch salad bars: not everything is good for your diet. Avoid salads based on potatoes, pasta and rice, and never help yourself to one of the creamy dressings.

Food type	Carb (g)	Fibre (g)	Cal (kcal)	Pro (g)	Fat (g)
Chicken strips, portion	3	0.2	64	4.8	3.7
Chicken wings, portion	3	2.3	466	40	32.7
Fish					
Cod, in batter, fried	11.7	n/a	247	16.1	15.4
Fish and chips	43.5	3.9	465	27.5	20.1
Fish in a bun	62.8	3.4	510	34.2	13.5
Plaice, in batter, fried	12	n/a	257	15.2	16.8
Rock salmon/dogfish, in batter, fried	10.3	n/a	295	14.7	21.9
Skate, in batter, fried	4.9	n/a	168	14.7	10.1
Pizza/Pasta					
Cannelloni, per portion	38.7	n/a	556	20.9	35.4
Deep-pan pizza, per slice:					
Margherita	31.5	n/a	256	13.5	8.5
Meat Feast	28	n/a	266	13	11.3
Supreme	29.6	n/a	257	13.1	9.6
Vegetarian	14.8	n/a	136	6.9	5.6
Lasagne, per portion	62.4	9.3	669	39.4	29.2
Medium-pan pizza, per slice:					
Ham & Mushroom	34	n/a	269	13	10.2

TIP: If you're eating out, avoid any sauces made with flour. Ask the waiter; you won't be the first person to do so.

Food type	Carb (g)	Fibre (g)	Cal (kcal)	Pro (g)	Fat (g)
Medium-pan pizza, contd:					
Ham & Pineapple	28	1.3	241	12.1	8.9
Margherita	37.5	n/a	291	14.4	10.2
Meat Feast	27.8	n/a	324	16.6	16.2
Supreme	26.5	n/a	297	13.7	14.6
Vegetarian	26.2	1.8	225	10.5	8.8
Thin crust, per slice:					
Cheese & Tomato	18.2	1.7	126	6.7	2.9
Full House	18.9	1.3	183	9.3	7.8
Mixed Grill	19.6	1.7	177	9	6.9
Pepperoni	20.6	1.4	187	9	7.6
Tandoori Hot	18.7	1.9	138	8.2	3.5
Thin crust, per pizza:					
American	87.3	n/a	753	35.3	32.4
Fiorentina	88.4	n/a	740	38.22	27.5
Four Cheese	87.2	n/a	636	29.4	22.1
Ham & Mushroom	87.4	n/a	665	34.9	22.8
Mushroom	87.5	n/a	627	30.1	20.6
Tomato Bake, per portion	92.9	5.5	653	27.1	21.6
Tortellini, per portion	91.9	n/a	1116	26.9	71.3
Side Orders					
Fries, regular portion	28.3	2.8	206	2.9	9
Fries, large portion	33.3	2.4	550	36.2	30.3
Garlic bread, portion	55.4	n/a	407	10.1	16.1

Food type	Carb (g)	Fibre (g)	Cal (kcal)	Pro (g)	Fat (g)
Garlic bread with cheese, portion	43.2	n/a	587	31.3	32.2
Garlic mushrooms, portion	31.6	n/a	240	5.5	10.1
Hash browns	15.8	1.7	138	1.4	7.7
Potato skins, portion	32	n/a	571	36.2	34.2
Salade Niçoise, per portion	65	n/a	729	40	37
Drinks					
Milkshake, vanilla, regular, each	62.7	–	383	10.8	10.1
Dips					
BBQ Dip, portion	9.4	n/a	39	0.4	0.1
Cheesy Bites:					
Cheddar	28.7	n/a	319	8.5	18.9
Tomato & Cheddar	26.9	n/a	308	8.2	18.6
Garlic & Herb Dip, portion	6.21	n/a	280	1.29	27.75
Ranch Dip, portion	3.8	n/a	489	3.2	51
Meals					
All-day breakfast	46	3.7	715	30.3	49.5
Egg & chips	32.5	2.7	490	20.8	30.6

TIP: Chicken may be good for you, but chicken nuggets are bad for your diet, as is fried chicken. The coatings are usually based on breadcrumbs or flour, and they are normally deep-fried using lots of trans fats.

Food type	Carb (g)	Fibre (g)	Cal (kcal)	Pro (g)	Fat (g)
Mixed grill	46.4	3.9	770	36.7	49.1
Spicy Chicken Bake, portion	80.7	–	499	18.5	12.4
Sandwiches and Wraps					
Cheese & pickle, per pack	51	3.8	341	16	8.1
Cheese & tomato, per pack	42	4.4	288	20	4.6
Chicken & ham, per pack	34	3.2	294	25	6.4
Chicken salad wrap, per pack	22	1.7	152	9.4	3.1
Egg mayonnaise & cress,					
per pack	47	3.7	323	23	4.8
Egg salad, per pack	44	2	304	13	8.4
Flatbread:					
chicken tikka	24	0.7	172	11	3.6
Peking duck	29	1.9	169	7.4	2.6
spicy Mexican	24	1.9	153	8	2.7
tuna	19	1.3	123	8.8	1.3
Ham & Double Gloucester,					
per pack	35	4.5	307	20	9.7
Ham, cheese & pickle, per pack	33	5	296	22	8.4
Ham & cream cheese bagel,					
per pack	45	2.4	319	19	7
Mini sushi selection, per pack	53	4.1	293	9.6	4.7
Prawn mayonnaise, per pack	42	5	287	19	4.6
Roast chicken, per pack	32	6.5	297	28	6.6
Roast chicken salad, per pack	40	8.8	317	26	5.9

Food type	Carb (g)	Fibre (g)	Cal (kcal)	Pro (g)	Fat (g)
Salmon & cucumber, per pack	34	5.2	272	18	6.8
Toasted tea cake & butter	35.2	1.7	245	5.8	9.8
Tuna & cucumber, per pack	41	3.5	307	24	5.3
Tuna & sweetcorn, per pack	47	3.7	323	23	4
Tuna melt, per pack	33	2.6	258	21	4.7

TIP: When it comes to party food avoid cheese straws, sandwiches and crisps. Go for cocktail sausages (as long as they're not in a sweet sauce), nuts, chunks of cheese and any raw vegetables and fruit. Better still, eat before you go so you won't be so easily tempted.

Putting it into Practice

MENU IDEAS

All of the new high-protein diets have different 'rules and regulations', and while many of them have delicious recipes which conform to their guidelines, it is always good to do your own culinary thing sometimes. Use some of the following suggestions for inspiration, adapting them to the requirements of your particular diet.

Breakfast

- Fruit smoothie with a slice of wholegrain toast and Marmite
- Fresh fruit salad with natural yoghurt
- Mushrooms on toast
- High-fibre cereal with strawberries
- Scrambled eggs with mushrooms, tomato and chopped spinach
- Poached eggs and smoked haddock
- Kippers, garnished with chopped tomato
- Eggs Florentine – poached egg on a bed of chopped spinach
- Asparagus and mushroom omelette
- Smoked salmon frittata
- Central European continental breakfast – cold ham or other lean meat, slices of cheese, a hard-boiled egg and an orange

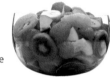

Lunch

- Chicken Caesar salad
- Tofu, herb and lemon dip with vegetable strips
- Borlotti bean and feta salad – mix cooked beans with sliced onion rings and half a tomato, chopped; crumble in the feta, dress with olive oil and a little lemon juice, and stir well
- Ham and cheese omelette with a green salad
- Chef's salad – cold turkey, cold roast beef and low-fat cheese on mixed leaves dressed with vinaigrette
- Celery and stilton soup
- Tuna and salad pitta – half a wholemeal pitta filled with a mixture of tinned tuna, sliced onion and red pepper, salad leaves and vinaigrette
- Stir-fried chicken with oriental vegetables, lemongrass and ginger
- Salad wraps – cos lettuce leaves rolled round one of the following options: cold meat spread with mustard; cream cheese with garlic and herbs; a mixture of chopped hard-boiled egg, mayo and a little paprika; guacamole; peanut butter and cream cheese.
- Spinach and bacon salad
- Smoked haddock soup

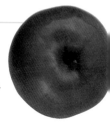

• Salade Niçoise – salad leaves, chopped tomato and green pepper, raw French beans, spring onions, cucumber, tuna, a hard-boiled egg and anchovies

Snacks

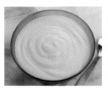

Some high-protein diets encourage snacks and others don't. If yours does not, then don't give into temptation. Here are some ideas if it does.

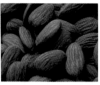

• A few olives
• 30 pistachios
• 30g of low-fat cheese
• A hard-boiled egg
• A small apple with 3-4 almonds

• 125g fat-free yoghurt
• 75g reduced-fat cottage cheese with half a chopped tomato
• Cheese dip with radishes
• Hummus with celery sticks
• No-fat Greek yoghurt with chopped almonds

Dinners

- Grilled salmon with roast Mediterranean vegetables
- Baked fish with tomato, red onion, basil, capers and a green salad
- Stir-fried chicken with broccoli and peppers
- Grilled goat's cheese on a large field mushroom, served on a bed of green salad with vinaigrette dressing
- Steak with mushroom sauce and mixed vegetables
- Grilled mackerel with lime and black pepper, served with green salad
- Prawns in garlic butter served on a cos lettuce salad
- Chilli baked beans, made using soya beans instead of the usual haricots and chilli powder (or a chopped fresh chilli) added to the tomato sauce

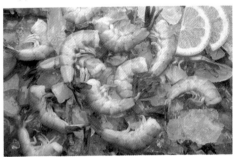

- Tandoori chicken with salad and a cucumber raita
- Grilled steak with garlic butter and French beans –
  press crushed peppercorns into the steak before
  cooking under the grill or on a ridged grill
  pan on top of the oven
- Marinated lamb kebabs with tsatsiki
  and a green salad
- Stir-fried tofu and vegetables –
  finely sliced mushrooms,
  onion, red pepper, mangetout,
  spring onions – with ginger,
  garlic and a little soy sauce

Desserts

Again, some high-protein diets allow desserts, and
others don't. Stick with whatever your diet recommends.

- Strawberry smoothie made by blending plenty of
  fruit with natural yoghurt
- Fresh fruit salad
- Poached pears in red wine
- Strawberries dipped in 70%-cocoa chocolate
- Fresh pear with 30g blue cheese and walnuts
- Baked apple
- Stewed rhubarb with cream
- Sliced melon medley – mix slices of
  different melon varieties and serve slightly chilled

- Ricotta and almonds
- Egg custards, flavoured with vanilla essence
- Frozen raspberry cream – blend double cream with still-frozen raspberries and serve at once
- Greek yoghurt topped with fresh berries and scattered with chopped roast hazelnuts

EATING OUT

Some of the high-protein diets are more flexible than others when it comes to eating out but it would be extremely difficult during any introductory phase. Here are some general guidelines which can help, and some specific suggestions for different cuisines.

- Read the whole menu before making your choice, and don't be afraid to ask questions.
- If you are offered bread while studying the menu, decline.
- Don't have any alcohol until you start eating, and then sip water as well.
- Soups are often a good choice but avoid creamy ones as they are often thickened with potato.
- Choose dishes which are grilled, steamed, stir-fried or poache, and avoid anything deep-fried, battered or in breadcrumbs.

- Avoid sauces made using flour – just ask. Check if any dressings contain sugar and, best of all, use oil and vinegar at the table.
- No chips or potatoes of any kind.
- Share a dessert if you can't resist, or have cheese (without the biscuits) or coffee instead. If you don't drink coffee, try mint tea which can be refreshing.

British

Go for food that has been simply cooked and have some extra vegetables or a side salad instead of potatoes. Use the Zone Diet's portion control shortcut: a third of your plate protein, the other two thirds non-starchy vegetables.

Choose:

- Kippers, smoked salmon, oysters
- Liver and bacon
- Grilled Dover sole or poached salmon
- Smoked haddock with a poached egg
- Grilled lean meat or fish
- Roast meat, but remove visible fat
- Grilled steak

Avoid:
· Bread and rolls
· Full English breakfast, which is high in saturated fat and often cooked in the 'wrong' fats
· Anything in batter or breadcrumbs
· Prepared meats like sausage or haggis
· Potatoes
· Pastry
· Yorkshire pudding
· Traditional puddings like spotted dick or rich ones like banoffi pie

Chinese

This is a difficult cuisine for anyone on a high-protein diet. Many of the sauces are high in carbs and the rice should be avoided; resist sharing other people's dishes. 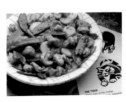 Monosodium glutamate (MSG), which is high in carbs, is often used as a thickening agent.

Choose:
· Clear soups without wontons or noodles
· Steamed, grilled or baked fish
· Stir-fried dishes without sauces

- Spare ribs but plain (no barbecue sauce)
- Steamed tofu dishes
- Stir-fried vegetables

Avoid:
- Rice
- Dim sum, wontons and spring rolls
- Sweet and sour dishes, and anything else with batter
- Sesame prawn toasts
- The pancakes with Peking or crispy duck
- Chow mein or other noodle dishes

French

Traditional French food might suit the Atkins Diet but most people will want to avoid those rich sauces. On the plus side, it is usually easy to find plain steaks or grilled fish but avoid the *frites* (chips). Omelettes are also often available.

Choose:
- Salads
- Consommé or French onion soup but without any bread
- Crudités – strips of raw vegetables
- *Moules* – mussels but check the sauce they are in fits your diet
- Grilled steak or fish

- Omelette and green salad
- *Fruits de mer* – seafood platter
- *Bouillabaisse* – fish stew/soup but no rouille sauce

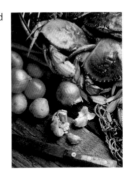

Avoid:
- Bread
- Croissants
- Rich sauces
- Creamy soups
- Potatoes in any form
- Pastry – quiches, anything *en croûte* (wrapped in pastry), fruit tarts
- *Crêpes* and *galettes*
- Rich desserts
- Patisserie and cakes

Greek

Greek food has plenty of options for anyone on a high-protein diet. There should be lots of plain grilled dishes to choose from, after you've eliminated any dishes with potatoes, pastry or rice. Beware the pitta bread that is often offered with starters but feel free to nibble on olives, carrot sticks and radishes. Note that 'Turkish' coffee often contains a lot of sugar.

Choose:
- Greek salad with cucumber, onion, feta, olives and tomato
- Hummus, taramasalata and tsatsiki with raw vegetables
- Grilled fish, seafood and meat, including kebabs
- *Stifatho* – beef casseroled with onions and tomatoes

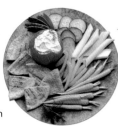

Avoid:
- Pitta bread
- *Dolmades* – vine leaves stuffed with rice
- *Spanakopitta* – a spinach and feta pie made with filo pastry
- *Gigantes pilaki* – a stew involving beans and other bean dishes
- Anything deep fried
- Moussaka
- Spicy sausages and meatballs because of the filler they contain
- Sweet puddings (that's most of them)

Indian

Indian food can be problematic. Curries aren't so satisfying without breads or rice and there are many problems lurking among the curries anyway. It's best to be careful and avoid getting into a situation where you're sharing dishes with other people who are not on a diet.

Choose:
- Tandoori dishes with salad and lemon, and tikkas but not tikka masala
- Raitas – chopped vegetable, often cucumber, and yoghurt
- Vegetables but not with potatoes
- Dishes involving *paneer* (cheese) but check sauces
- Any baked meat or fish dishes
- Fresh fruit, not fruit canned in syrup

Avoid:
- Deep-fried, battered starters or ones with pastry such as samosas or pakora
- All breads
- Rice
- Dishes with thick sauces and those containing chick-peas or beans
- Dhals
- Thick, sweetened chutneys
- Potato dishes
- All Indian desserts and ice creams; tinned fruit in syrup

Italian

Pizzas and pasta aren't the be-all and end-all of Italian cooking and following high-protein guidelines should be comparatively easy. Desserts are a different story unless there's fresh fruit so stick to coffee; it should be excellent.

Choose:

- Antipasti – figs or melon with Parma ham; cold meats, grilled vegetables, olives, etc.
- Thin soups but not if they contain pasta
- Salads, including *tricolore* – tomato, mozzarella and avocado
- Grilled fish, poultry or meat
- Stewed or casseroled meat and fish dishes (but check with the waiter that there's no flour in the sauce)
- Meat escalopes but not coated in breadcrumbs
- Fresh fruit

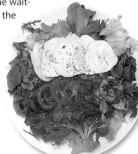

Avoid:

- Bread of all kinds
- Pasta
- Pizza
- Risotto

- Polenta, which is made with maize flour
- Anything deep-fried like seafood
- Rich, sticky desserts and ice cream

Japanese

There are many high-protein pitfalls in Japanese restaurants, perhaps surprisingly given the popularity of fish and tofu. Avoiding rice, noodles, batter and rice wrappers can be difficult, so ask questions. On the plus side, the flavourings are excellent: soy sauce, wasabi (strong horseradish) and sesame oil are common.

Choose:
- Tofu dishes but not deep-fried ones
- *Teppanyaki* – plain grilled fish or meat with vegetables
- Sashimi – raw fresh fish with wasabi
- Steamed fish or poultry
- *Shabu-shabu* – thin slices of beef quickly cooked in stock, with vegetables

Avoid:
- Rice including many types of sushi, and noodles
- *Tempura* – food in batter, usually vegetables

- Teriyaki sauce, high in carbs from sugar
- Anything in a rice wrapper
- Anything coated in breadcrumbs and fried
- *Mirin* (sweetened saké) or *miso* (fermented soya beans) in dishes

Mexican

Mexican food is a minefield if you're on a high-protein diet but stick with the plainest food possible and you should be all right. Rice and bread are off-limits and you're not allowed tortillas either.

Choose:

- Guacamole with raw vegetables
- Tomato salsa
- Grilled fish, meat or poultry
- Salads
- *Ceviche* – raw fish salad with avocado
- Chicken wings

Avoid:

- Anything involving tortillas or tacos
- Rice
- Heavy sauces
- Nachos
- Chilli con carne
- Refried beans

- *Torta* – filled sandwiches and rolls
- Any pastries or desserts

Middle Eastern

There should be plenty of grilled food on a Middle Eastern menu, both meat and fish. However, this cuisine also uses a lot of pulses and those may be off-limits. Sticky puddings are out, of course, and the coffee will probably be automatically prepared with sugar unless you specifically ask for filter coffee.

Choose:
- *Baba ghanoush* – an aubergine dip – with raw vegetables
- *Gibneh beyda* – white cheese (usually feta) dip
- Grilled meat or fish
- Kebabs
- Most salads except *tabbouleh*
- *Kofta* – minced meat on skewers

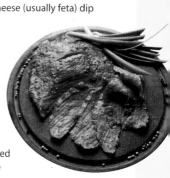

Avoid:
- Rice and couscous
- Bread
- *Kibbeh*, made with cracked wheat and minced lamb

- *Tabbouleh*, a salad made with bulgar wheat
- Stuffed vegetables, as rice is usually the stuffing
- Pastries, savoury and sweet
- Rich desserts
- *Lokhoum* – 'Turkish delight'

Spanish

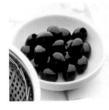

Grilled food is often on the menu in Spanish restaurants, but many classic Spanish dishes are impossible – no paella, for instance. Chorizo and other sausages may contain filler which would take them off the list too.

Choose:

- Olives and nuts
- Salads
- White anchovies in vinegar (*boccarones*)
- *Escalivada* – roasted vegetable salad
- *Zarzuela* – a seafood stew
- Gazpacho – cold soup made with tomatoes and peppers but avoid croûtons
- Grilled meats, fish and seafood
- Any omelettes that don't contain potatoes (avoid *tortilla español*)

Avoid:

- Rice dishes, including paella
- Anything deep-fried including *churros* – strips of dough
- Chorizo and other prepared meats
- Dishes including potatoes or pulses
- *Flan caramelo* – caramel custard
- Pastries
- Rich desserts
- *Turron* – nougat

Thai

No rice or noodles, of course, which may give you problems. Thai red and green curries are often made with coconut milk, which should be fine as far as high-protein diets are concerned despite the fact that they are rather high in calories. The same applies to meat or chicken satay.

Choose:

- *Tom yam* soup – a clear soup with chicken or fish and vegetables
- Salads, often with beef or fish
- Stir-fried meat and seafood
- Green and red curries
- Steamed fish, seafood or tofu dishes
- Chicken or meat satay
- Fresh fruits

Avoid:
- Rice
- Noodles
- Dishes with rice or noodles like *pho*, a soup
- Spring rolls
- Crab cakes with sugary chilli sauce
- Anything deep-fried

Packed meals

Most of us regularly eat away from home – particularly when we're at work. Think seriously about taking a packed lunch as staff restaurants, sandwich bars and coffee shops are packed with pitfalls. If you are following a diet which permits some bread then you may want to use your bread allowance to make a sandwich. However, think about alternatives like salads or soup (invest in a wide-mouthed flask just for soup) or chicken drumsticks.

If your diet allows it, take fruit. You may also need some snacks, again depending on your diet, so take olives or a few pistachios. Avoid sugary carbonated drinks, boxes of fruit juice and flavoured mineral water as they all contain too much sugar.

Possible toppings for bread:
- Smoked salmon and chopped dill pickle

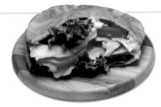

- Hard-boiled egg, chopped and mixed with mayo and black pepper
- Low-fat cream cheese blended with tuna and some chopped onion
- Cold meat with tomatoes
- Low-fat cottage cheese and lettuce leaves
- A quick pâté made by blending smoked mackerel fillets with cream cheese and a little lemon juice

Salads

- Cold turkey, beansprouts, spring onions and mangetout, with a dressing made from soy sauce and lemon juice
- Strips of raw vegetables plus radishes and cauliflower florets with a feta cheese and low-fat natural yoghurt dip
- Smoked fish or cold meat in chunks, grated carrot, shredded cabbage and spring onions, dressed with a little olive oil and lime juice
- Pieces of cold chicken, tomato, onion rings, olives on a bed of lettuce leaves

- Baby spinach leaves together with baby beet leaves, dressed with oil and vinegar and with cold bacon crumbled over the top (take the bacon separately or it will go soggy)
- Smoked mackerel, flaked, with radishes and strong-tasting salad leaves like rocket; add a little horseradish to the dressing

Soups (preferably homemade):
- Thai fish soup
- Aubergine, tomato and garlic soup
- Mushroom soup (with some lentils if your diet permits)
- Chicken and Chinese mushroom soup
- Smoked haddock soup
- Tomato and basil soup

Avoid:
- Confectionery
- Crisps and similar snacks
- Biscuits and cakes
- Any fried food and sandwiches other than your own
- Coffee-shop cappuccinos and other very milky coffees – think of the carbs in all that milk

FURTHER READING

General Advice on Nutrition

Collins Gem Calorie Counter, HarperCollins, 2005

Collins Gem Carb Counter, HarperCollins, 2004

Collins Gem Healthy Eating, HarperCollins, 1999

Collins Gem What Diet? HarperCollins, 2005

Daily Telegraph Encyclopedia of Vitamins, Minerals & Herbal Supplements, Dr Sarah Brewer, Robinson, 2002

Fat is a Feminist Issue, Susie Orbach, Arrow, 1998

Fats That Heal, Fats That Kill, Udo Erasmus, Alive, 1998

Food Pharmacy, Jean Carper, Pocket Books, 2000

Good Fat, Bad Fat: Lower Your Cholesterol and Reduce Your Odds of a Heart Attack, P. Castelli, Glen C. Griffin, 1997

New 8-Week Cholesterol Cure, Robert E. Kowalski, HarperCollins, 2001

Nutrients A to Z, A User's Guide, Michael Sharon, Carlton Books, 2005, new edn

Optimum Nutrition Bible, Patrick Holdford, Piatkus, 1998

Prescription for Nutritional Healing, Phyllis and James F. Balch, Avery Publishing Inc, 2002

Bodyfoods for Busy People, Jane Clark, Quadrille, 2004

Eat, Drink, and be Healthy, Walter C Willet, MD, Simon & Schuster, 2001

L is for Label: How to Read Between the Lines on Food Packaging, Amanda Ursell, Hay House, 2004

Vitamins and Minerals Handbook, Sara Rose, Hamlyn, 2003

The CSIRO Diet

The CSIRO Total Wellbeing Diet, Dr Manny Noakes, Dr
   Peter Clifton, Penguin, 2005

The Atkins Diet

All books by Dr Robert C. Atkins
Dr Atkins' New Diet Revolution, Vermilion, 2003
Dr Atkins' Quick and Easy New Diet Cookbook, Pocket
   Books, 2003
Atkins for Life: the Next Level, Macmillan, 2003
*Dr Atkins Vita-Nutrient Solution: Nature's Answer to
   Drugs*, Pocket Books, 2003

The New High Protein Diet

All books by Charles Clark
The New High-Protein Diet, Vermilion, 2002
The New High-Protein Diet Cookbook, Charles Clark
   and Maureen Clark, Vermilion, 2002

The South Beach Diet

All books by Dr Arthur Agatston
The South Beach Diet, Headline, 2003
The South Beach Diet Cookbook, Random House, 2004

Vegetarian High-Protein Diets

The Vegetarian Low-Carb Diet, Rose Elliot, Piatkus,
   2005

The Zone
All books by Barry Sears, PhD
The Zone Diet, Thorsons, 1999
Mastering the Zone, HarperNewYork, 1997
A Week in the Zone, Harper Paperbacks, 2000
The Soy Zone, HarperCollins, 2001

Other High-protein Diet and Recipe Books
500 Low-Carb Recipes, Dana Carpenden, Fair Winds
    Press, 2002
The Complete Scarsdale Medical Diet, Herman Tarnower,
    MD and Samm Sinclair Baker, Bantam Books, 1995
The Formula: A Personalized 40-30-30 Fat-Burning, Gene
    and Joyce Doust, Ballantine Books, 2001
The Good Carb Cookbook, Sandra C. Woodruff, Avery
    Publishing Group, 2001
The Carbohydrate Addicts' Diet, Drs Rachael and Richard
    F. Heller, Vermilion, 2000
The Carbohydrate Addict's Calorie Counter, Drs Rachael
    and Richard F. Heller, Signet, 2000
The Carbohydrate Addict's Healthy Heart Programme,
    Drs Rachael and Richard F. Heller, Vermilion, 1998
Lose Weight the Smart Low-Carb Way, Bettina Newman
    and David Joachim, Rodale Books, 2002
The Low-Carb Comfort Food Cookbook, Michael R.
    Eades, John Wiley & Sons, 2003
The No-Grain Diet, Joseph Mercola, Hodder, 2004

Protein Power: The High Protein, Low-Carbohydrate Way to Lose Weight, Feel Fit and Boost Your Health, Michael R. Eades and Dr Mary Dan Eades, HarperCollins, 2000

PICTURE CREDITS

Photos copyright © Getty Images:
Michael Lamotte/Cole Group pp. 14, 39, 45(b), 51, 56, 58, 86, 142, 206, 217, 220, 230; Dennis Gray/Cole Group pp. 17, 54, 90, 128, 214, 216 (t), 216 (b); Ed Carey/Cole Group pp. 22, 49, 96; D.Fischer and P. Lyons/Cole Group pp. 23; Chris Shorten/Cole Group p. 42; Jackson Vereen/Cole Group pp. 45 (t), 47, 62, 130, 223; Kevin Sanchez/Cole Group pp. 78, 158, 166, 190, 221; Keith Ovregaard/Cole Group pp. 82, 168, 224; Victor Budnik/Cole Group pp. 136, 229; Bob Montesclaros/Cole Group pp. 148, 164, 233; Patricia Brabant/Cole Group pp. 184, 200, 218; Joel Glenn/Cole Group p. 227

Photos copyright © Photodisc: pp. 10, 25, 28, 35, 37, 104, 114, 156, 216 (c)

Photos by Christina Jansen, copyright © Grapevine Publishing Services: pp. 8, 19, 60, 63, 72, 120, 176, 182, 215, 226

USEFUL ADDRESSES

British Dietetic Association
5th Floor, Charles House
148/9 Great Charles Street
Queensway
Birmingham B3 3HT
www.bda.uk.com

British Heart Foundation
14 Fitzhardinge Street
London W1H 6DH
020 7935 0185

British Nutrition Foundation
High Holborn House
52-54 High Holborn
London WC1V 6RQ
020 7404 6504

Diabetes UK
10 Parkway
London NW1 7AA
Careline 0845 1202960
Or 020 7424 1000 and
ask for the Careline

Coronary Prevention Group
020 7927 2125
www.healthnet.org

Institute for Optimum Nutrition
Blades Court, Deodar Road
London SW15 2NU
020 8877 9993
No nutrition advice
given but they will
recommend a nutritionist

Women's Health Concern
PO Box 2126
Marlow
Bucks SL7 2PU
Tel. 0845 1232319 to
speak to a nurse
or 01628 488065 for other
information
www.womens-health-concern.org

USEFUL WEBSITES

www.charlesclark.uk.com
www.lowcarb.ca
www.southbeachdiet.com
www.low-carb-diet-recipes.com
www.bodyfoods.com
www.weightlossresources.co.uk
www.ivillage.co.uk (the Tesco website for diet
queries)
www.healthnet.org.uk (Coronary Prevention Group)
www.sainsburys.com/healthyeating
www.asda.com
www.edietsuk.co.uk (also used by Tesco)
www.weightlossresources.co.uk